THE INTERPROFESSIONAL
HEALTH CARE
TEAM

LEADERSHIP AND DEVELOPMENT

Donna Weiss, PhD, OTR/L, FAOTA
Associate Professor, Emeritus
Occupational Therapy Program
Department of Rehabilitation Sciences
College of Health Professions and Social Work
Temple University
Philadelphia, PA

Felice J. Tilin, PhD
Program Director
Graduate Organization Development and Leadership
Saint Joseph's University
Philadelphia, PA
President
GroupWorks Consulting, LLC
Narberth, PA

Marlene J. Morgan, EdD, OTR/L
Assistant Professor
The University of Scranton
Scranton, PA

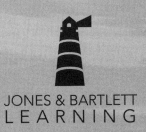

JONES & BARTLETT
LEARNING

World Headquarters
Jones & Bartlett Learning
5 Wall Street
Burlington, MA 01803
978-443-5000
info@jblearning.com
www.jblearning.com

Jones & Bartlett Learning books and products are available through most bookstores and online booksellers. To contact Jones & Bartlett Learning directly, call 800-832-0034, fax 978-443-8000, or visit our website, www.jblearning.com.

Production Credits

Publisher: William Brottmiller
Senior Acquisitions Editor: Katey Birtcher
Editorial Assistant: Sean Fabery
Production Manager: Julie Champagne Bolduc
Production Editor: Joanna Lundeen
Marketing Manager: Grace Richards
Manufacturing and Inventory Control Supervisor: Amy Bacus
Cover Designer: Michael O'Donnell
Composition: Publishers' Design and Production Services, Inc.
Cover, Title Page, and Front Matter Opener Image © AbleStock
Printing and Binding: Edwards Brothers Malloy
Cover Printing: Edwards Brothers Malloy

To order this product, use ISBN: 978-1-4496-7336-9

Library of Congress Cataloging-in-Publication Data
Weiss, Donna (Donna F.)
 The interprofessional health care team : leadership and development / by Donna Weiss, Felice J. Tilin, and Marlene J. Morgan.
  p. ; cm.
 Includes bibliographical references and index.
 ISBN 978-1-4496-2657-0 — ISBN 1-4496-2657-2
 I. Tilin, Felice J. II. Morgan, Marlene J. III. Title.
 [DNLM: 1. Patient Care Team—organization & administration. 2. Leadership. W 84.8]
 610.68—dc23
                                                                           2012039290
6048

Printed in the United States of America
17 16 15 14 13   10 9 8 7 6 5 4 3 2 1

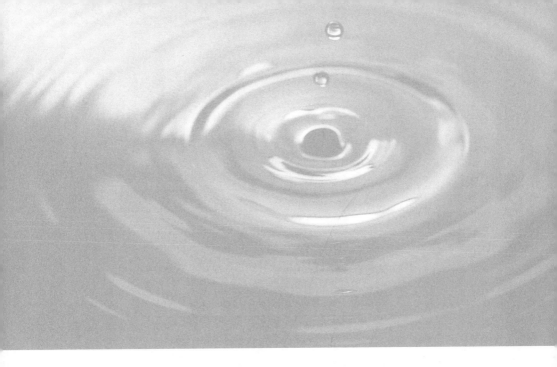

*To my husband, Leigh, for his optimism, energy,
and love and my granddaughter, Madeline Paige
Broome, for her wide-eyed wonder.*

— Donna Weiss

*To my spouse, Trudi Sippola, for all of her unwavering
support and to my loving parents, Sonya Tilin and in
memory of my father Edward Tilin, who both taught
me that developing relationships is the secret to a
happy and healthy life.*

— Felice J. Tilin

*To the memory of my parents, Al and Alice Morgan.
What more can I say?*

— Marlene J. Morgan

Contents

Preface   *ix*

Acknowledgments   *xiii*

About the Authors   *xv*

Reviewers   *xvii*

*Introduction: Interprofessional Leadership in
the Health Care Environment*   *xxi*

PART I   **Team and Group Development**   **1**

Chapter 1   **Groups-Teams-Systems**   **3**

Why Groups?   3

What Distinguishes a Group from a Random
Collection of People?   5

What Is the Difference Between a Team and
a Group?   5

A Systems Approach to Groups   7

Applying Systems Theory   10

Chapter 2   Group Development   **19**

The Group   19

What You See Is Not What You Get:
The Unconscious Life of a Group   22

Stages of Group Development   23

An Integrated Model of Group Development   26

Identifying the Stages of Group Development:
Characteristics and Goals   27

How Does the Stage of the Group Impact Team
Productivity?   33

Group Size: Less Is More   34

How Long Does It Take for a Group to Develop
Through Each Stage?   36

**Chapter 3   Team Building Blocks: Norms, Goals, Roles,
                Communication, Leaders, and Members**   **39**

Norms   39

Goals   41

Roles   42

Communication Patterns   46

Part I   Team and Group Development Activities   **61**

Activity 1: How Much of a Team Is Your Group?   63

Activity 2: *I* and *We*   63

Activity 3: TOPS: Team Orientation and
Performance Survey   63

Activity 4: Team Goal Setting   66

PART II   Relationship-Centered Leadership   **69**

Chapter 4   Perspectives on Leadership   **71**

Perspectives on Leadership   72

Personality and Trait Theories   72

Contingency and Situational Theories and
Leadership Styles   79
Relational Theories   82
Emotional Intelligence   82
Resonance   87

Chapter 5   Leadership Building Blocks   93

Power   94
Motivation   97
Learning   100

Chapter 6   Relational Leadership   109

The Leader as Learner   111
The Leader as Coach   112
The Leader as Partner   114
The Leader as Catalyst   114
The Leader as Ecologist   115

**Part II   Relationship-Centered Leadership
               Activities   121**

Activity 1: Myers-Briggs—Your Leadership Behavior
Under Stress and at Your Best   123
Activity 2: Best Manager   125
Activity 3: Leadership Learning Journey   126

**PART III Building and Sustaining Collaborative
            Interprofessional Teams   135**

Chapter 7   Leveraging Diversity   137

Surface-Level Diversity   139
Deep-Level Diversity   139
Integrating the Levels of Diversity   139

Managing Conflict 145

Chapter 8   Facilitating a Collaborative Culture 153

Facilitating a Collaborative Culture 153

Dr. Mary Sinnott, PT, DPT 158

Dr. Tim Fox, PT, DPT, GCS, and
Dr. Robyn Kurilko, PT, DPT 163

Sue Carol Verrillo, RN, MSN 167

Dr. Emily Keshner, PT, EdD 172

John J. Kirby, OTR/L, MBA 176

Rebecca Austill-Clausen, MS, OTR/L, FAOTA 181

Chapter 9   Generative Practices 187

Heal Thyself: The Importance of Personal Renewal 189

Affirmative Dialogue 191

Reframing 193

The Team as Learner 195

**Part III   Building and Sustaining Collaborative
Interprofessional Teams Activities 207**

Activity 1: Mini 360-Degree Feedback Exercise 209

Activity 2: The Art of Culture 209

Activity 3: Checklist of Behaviors That Foster
a Collaborative Culture 210

Index 213

Preface

Afaf Meleis, PhD, FAAN, DrPS (hon)
Margaret Bond Simon
Dean of the University
of Pennsylvania School of Nursing

Quality health care requires teamwork. Putting individuals together to teach across disciplines or to provide healthcare never guarantees the creation of a team with the synergy needed for a shared vision, an agreed upon mission, and a system of collaboration. To form productive and efficient teams requires a knowledge base, the use of best practices, interprofessional leadership, and individuals who are well prepared to be collaborative and effective members of the team.

It has become apparent, as evidenced in many policy reports and through much research, that teamwork is the hallmark of positive outcomes for the health and wellbeing of patients, families, and communities. Collaboration and partnership are equally as important and must be forged within and between organizations to advance well-being and enable institutions to function at their full capacities. However, it also has become apparent through many thoughtful dialogues and reports such as the *Health Professionals for a New Century: Transforming Education to Strengthen Health Systems in an Interdependent World*, written by the independent Lancet Commission on Education of Health

Professionals for the 21st Century, and *The Initiative on the Future of Nursing*, authored by the Institute of Medicine (IOM) Committee on behalf of the Robert Wood Johnson Foundation, that partnership, collaboration, and the formation of teams requires a paradigm shift in educational programs as well as in institutional function (Bhutta, Chen, Cohen et. al, 2010 and IOM, 2011).

Paradigm shifts occur through deliberate and systematic dialogues and debates. Productive dialogues and debates depend on knowledge of a field, willing participants, environments that promote such dialogues, diversity of opinions, respect of different voices, and trust in the value and principles that promote partnership and collaboration. Whether this paradigm shift is needed for crossing the boundaries of professions and developing interprofessional education, moving the silos of different disciplines toward interdisciplinarity or the ethos of independence toward interdependence, it fundamentally depends upon and requires the use of a well-organized and comprehensive evidence-based knowledge foundation and tools for implementation.

This book provides the much-needed knowledge base for developing a relational leadership style that promotes interdisciplinarity, interprofessionalism, and productive teamwork. It describes possibilities and options, theories, exercises, rich references, and stimulating questions that will inspire both novices and experts to think differently about their roles and styles as leaders or members of a team. I venture to suggest that this book will become a very important resource that will lead to more constructive actions for the development of a collaborative culture. The authors provide many tools to empower readers and facilitate the fostering of productive teamwork. It is an inspiring book with easily operational principles. My gratitude goes out to the authors for having the wisdom, the knowledge, and the experience to invest in writing this book. As teaching faculty members, students, clinicians, leaders, and managers read it and discuss its ideas, they will be as grateful to the authors as I have been after reviewing and using its content. It is written for many audiences and to achieve many goals all centered on best practices to attain quality care, particularly during this time of reinventing and transforming health care.

References

Bhutta, Z.A., Chen, L., Cohen, J., Crisp, N., Evans, T., Fineberg, H., Frenk, J., Garcia, P., Horton, R., Ke, Y., Kelley, P., Kistnasamy, B., Meleis, A.I., Naylor, D., Pablos-Mendez, A., Reddy, S., Scrimshaw, S., Sepulveda, J., Serwadda, D., Zurayk, H. (2010). Education of health professionals for the 21st century: A global independent commission. *The Lancet, 375*(9721), 1137–38.

IOM (Institute of Medicine). 2011. *The Future of Nursing: Leading Change, Advancing Health.* Washington, DC: The National Academies Press.

Acknowledgments

Our individual contributions to this book are products of the innumerable relationships that we have been fortunate enough to enjoy over the course of our professional and personal lives. Through our collaboration on this book, we have been edified and transformed by the experiences of each other. We share the deepest gratitude for the thought, guidance and support that we have received from the following people:

To mentors: Susan A. Wheelan, Annie McKee, and Sherene Zolno who generously shared their scholarship and fostered our learning.

To colleagues, teachers, clients, friends, and family for sharing their stories and wisdom: Rebecca Austill-Clausen, Stephen Berg, Marco Bertola, Joanne Broder Summerson, Luis Constantino, Claire Conway, Wanda Cooper, Laurie Cousart, Vincent Curren, Dan Drake, Mario DiCioccio, Peter Doukas, Tim Fox, Kevin Hook, Francis Johnston, Emily Keshner, Moya Kinnealey, John Kirby, Robin Kurilko, Delores Mason, Karen Nichols, Eileen Sullivan-Marx, Afaf Meleis, Linda Paolini, Prem Rawat, Melanie Rothschild, Carol L. Savrin, Stephen Scardina, Judith Shamian, Carole Simon, Mary Sinnott, Beth Sippola, Rob Sippola, Trudi

Sippola, David M. Smith, Bruce Theriault, Kelsey Tilin, Sam Tilin, Beulah Trey, and Sue Carol Verrillo.

To the team at Jones & Bartlett Learning who patiently provided support, advice, and encouragement throughout the publication process: Katey Birtcher, Teresa Reilly, Sean Fabery, and Joanna Lundeen.

Special thanks are extended to Felice's colleagues at Saint Joseph's University who provided the time and encouragement to complete this book: Karin Botto, Jeanne Brady, Sabrina DeTurk, William Madges, Robert Palestini, Becky Rice, Erin Schwing, and Wendy Thruman.

Finally, we acknowledge all learners—whether they are students, teachers, leaders, or group members—and their active engagement in asking questions and trying on new ways of thinking, being, and doing.

About the Authors

Donna Weiss, PhD, OTR/L, FAOTA is a coach, trainer and facilitator in the areas of interpersonal communication, group dynamics and leadership.

Felice J. Tilin, PhD is an organization development consultant, facilitator, executive coach, and educator with multinational, private and non-profit businesses and healthcare organizations in the US, Canada, Europe, Africa and Asia.

Marlene J. Morgan, EdD, OTR/L has extensive experience in clinical and academic leadership positions and her research interests include interdisciplinary education for health professionals.

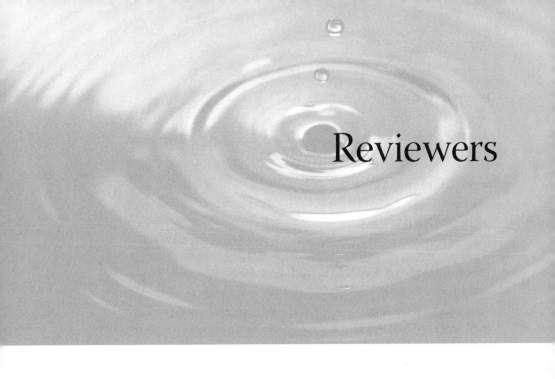

Reviewers

Patrick C. Auth, PhD, PA-C
Chair
Physician Assistant Department
Drexel University
Philadelphia, PA

Linda C. Caplis, MS, RT(R)
Clinical Assistant Professor
Towson University
Towson, MD

Joy Doll, OTD
Assistant Professor
Director
Post-Professional OTD Program
Creighton University
Omaha, NE

Cristina Dumitrescu, MS, OTR/L
Associate Director and Assistant Professor
Academic Fieldwork Coordinator
Mercy College
Dobbs Ferry, NY

Deborah A. Greenawald, PhD, RN, CNE
Associate Professor
Alvernia University
Reading, PA

Jaime S. Greene, MS, EMT-B
President/CEO
Safety Associates, Inc.
Greenacres, FL

Deborah Giedosh, EdD, MS-Ned, MS, BSN, RN
Director of Nursing
Alaska Career College
Anchorage, AK

Margaret Gillingham, MS
Lecturer
University of Baltimore
Baltimore, MD

Jason Glowczewski, PharmD, MBA
Manager of Pharmacy and Oncology
University Hospitals Geauga Medical Center
Chardon, OH
Affiliate Assistant Professor of Pharmacy Practice
Findlay University
Findlay, OH

Lauren R. Goodloe, PhD, RN, NEA-BC
Director of Medical and Geriatric Nursing
Administrative Director for Research
Assistant Dean for Clinical Operations
Virginia Commonwealth University School of Nursing
Richmond, VA

Tina Gunaldo, PT, DTP, MHS
Instructor
Louisiana State University Health Sciences Center
New Orleans, LA

Wilton Kennedy, MMS, DHSc, PA-C
Director of Clinical Education
Jefferson College of Health Sciences
Roanoke, VA

Judi Schack-Dugre, PT, DPT, MBA
Instructor
University of Central Florida
Orlando, FL

Introduction: Interprofessional Leadership in the Health Care Environment

Learning Objectives

1. Understand the interprofessional health care team as a broadly inclusionary concept.
2. Describe how an interprofessional orientation can enhance patient care.
3. Explain the importance of relationship-centered care to patient outcomes.
4. Understand the concept of members as leaders.

Human beings are social by nature and bond together in families, small groups, and tribes. As we attempt to navigate from childhood through adulthood, our behaviors tend to mirror those of our family groups, peer groups, and professional groups. As we mature, our sense of self is created, in part, by our interactions with and feedback from these groups. Over the millennia, interaction with a variety of other people has been necessary to fulfill primary needs like love and affection but also to accomplish the work inherent to community building and survival. With the evolution of societies from the Stone Age through the Information Age, the complexity of the challenges that individuals and organizations face has increased, as well as the need for well-functioning, diverse groups who can meet those challenges. Solving complex problems requires diverse information sets that are not the purview of a single person or a single profession. This is true in all modern endeavors but most apparent in the healthcare industry.

The concept of health incorporates a complex and holistic system where biological, psychological, physical, socioeconomic, cultural, and environmental factors function as interconnected and interacting determinants of one another. Rowe (2003) has noted that health issues are characteristically broad and complex and are most appropriately examined from an interdisciplinary perspective. Reports from the Pew Health Professions Commission (1998), the Institutes of Medicine (2001, 2002, 2003), and the World Health Organization (WHO, 2010) have repeatedly supported the notion that educational programs for health professionals can only be considered complete if they include experiences working in interdisciplinary teams. The literature regarding higher education is replete with references to research, as well as, interdisciplinary, interprofessional, and integrative studies. External funding sources for research identify evidence of interdisciplinary collaboration as a key criterion for grant eligibility (Bray, Adamson, & Mason, 2007; García & Roblin, 2008; Palincsar, 2007). Evidence of interdisciplinary team experiences is included in the accreditation standards for many health professional education programs with the expectation that health professionals will be educated with an interdisciplinary orientation and will develop an ability to leverage the power of teams to solve complex problems (Frenk et al., 2010; IPEC Report, 2011; NIH, 2008; Royeen, Jensen, & Harvan, 2009).

Members of interdisciplinary healthcare teams have multiple reporting relationships and value systems. Finding themselves working in increasingly complex organizational and political structures. The competitive healthcare market presents professionals with a variety of leadership challenges—not the least of which is learning to leverage the power of interdisciplinarity. Drinka and Clark (2000) define an interdisciplinary healthcare team (IHCT) as "a group of individuals with diverse training and backgrounds who work together as an identified unit or system" (p.6). Disciplinary expertise is maximized when members of the interdisciplinary healthcare team can routinely employ strong relational skills and effectively coordinate their work with others. Relational coordination in the form of high-quality communication, mutual positive regard, trust, and active engagement are associated with a stronger collective identity, reduction in status differential, increased ability to respond to pressures with resilience, job satisfaction, and retention of staff. Most importantly, organizations that institutionalize the consistent communication strategies associated with relationship-centered organizations are high performing and profitable, demonstrating low employee turnover, better clinical outcomes, reduction in length of stay, and enhanced patient-perceived quality care (Gittell, 2009; Suchman, Sluyter, & Williamson, 2011).

The trend toward specialization in the health professions may lead to a less inclusionary interpretation of Drinka and Clark's definition of interdisciplinarity. It may be interpreted as the inclusion of persons who have the same basic training but have a specialty. For instance, some people may consider an internist, gynecologist, and a physiatrist to be an interdisciplinary team. The term *interprofessional* connotes a broader perspective and may include persons who have professional licensure or certification in nursing, occupational therapy, physical therapy, speech and language pathology, social work, and other health-related professions in addition to physicians (Hammock, Freeth, Copperman, & Goodsman, 2009). In literature and in practice, the terms are often used interchangeably.

Health care evolved from a hierarchical process dominated by physicians to an inclusionary team of professionals. Recently, the team was broadened to include patients and caregivers. The conceptual shift regarding the focus of health care occurred in tandem with the recognition of health care as a complex system of relationships. Neither term—*interdisciplinary* nor *interprofessional*—reflects the importance of the patient and other important constituencies/contexts in the achievement of good patient outcomes. The more cogent term seems to be *relationship-centered*.

The notion of relationship-centered healthcare teams reaches beyond the traditional core of physicians, nurses, and therapists; it incorporates all the constituencies who impact patient outcomes. It implies that the construction of healthcare teams is unique to the individual patient needs. The breakdown of traditional professional boundaries is necessary to meet the challenge of providing quality and cost-effective health care that is accessible to increasing populations (Grant & Finocchio, 1995). Skills in team building, team membership, and the understanding of the group dynamics are foundational and indispensable for the next generation of healthcare leaders.

Whether teams are called interdisciplinary, interprofessional, or relationship centered, each member of the healthcare team needs to ask these important questions:

- Who needs to be involved in order for the best patient outcomes to be achieved?
- How can we work together to achieve those outcomes efficiently and effectively?
- What is my unique professional and personal contribution to the team?
- How can I facilitate the optimum functioning of the team and the best client outcomes?

The full potential of the interprofessional healthcare team is realized when each member assumes a leadership stance. The member as a leader recognizes the power of his/her unique professional expertise and personal qualities. He/she accepts the responsibility of actively contributing relationship-centered, safe, effective, and quality health services. The designated leader is responsible for drawing out the leadership stance in all team members by modeling self-awareness, self-regulation, empathy, and positive communication and encouraging these behaviors in others (Boyatzis & McKee, 2005). Leaders who are successful in facilitating a proactive leadership stance throughout their teams realize that their own perspective is incomplete and recognize the value of engaging the wisdom and power of the collective. In doing so, they create sustainable, relationship-centered, and highly productive team cultures that are creatively resilient in the face of change and thrive over time.

Leadership in the interprofessional healthcare team means that both the designated leader and members must be willing to share the responsibilities of team leadership and be cognizant of group dynamics in order to work with widely diverse skills, values, and interests (Lee, 2010). Appropriately addressing these issues requires a strong leadership that has a broad and integrative perspective. The leadership should be embraced by a cadre of professionals who leverage their own disciplinary knowledge base and integrate it with those of other related disciplines in order to develop advanced understanding and competence in patient-centered and relationship-centered practice. The accountability for this type of leadership is shared by health professionals at all organizational levels who engage in research, teaching, health administration, and health policy development, as well as direct patient care.

The challenge that faces health professionals is that while most health professionals work in interprofessional teams and recognize their value, the majority have been professionally acculturated into their respective professional guilds rather than seeing themselves as members of an interprofessional team. Until recently, professional training in most of the health disciplines did not emphasize collaboration, group decision making, or shared leadership (Calhoun et al., 2008; Lee, 2010). The Institutes of Medicine reported that a lack of effective collaboration among disciplines was most often identified as the cause of medical errors (IOM, 1999, 2003). For example, a boy dies of a treatable infection or pain reducing palliative care is withheld from a terminally ill patient for want of interprofessional collaboration (Dowd, 2012; Brown, 2012). On the other hand, effective interprofessional collaboration is linked to improved patient outcomes (Wheelan, Burchill, & Tilin, 2003). "It is becoming increasingly apparent the effort to produce high quality care is not hampered by lack of clinical expertise in the individual professions but rather by lack of appropriate knowledge and experience among these groups as to how to make these multidisciplinary teams work well" (Freshman, Rubino, & Chassiakos, 2010, p. 6).

As health systems increase in complexity, health professionals need to develop confidence in group problem solving, successful conflict management and resolution, efficient and effective information exchange, and boundary management (Gray, 2008). These competencies are dependent upon an understanding of the stages of group development and what makes teams effective. An effective team shows high levels of reflectivity and self-management skill, the ability to develop and maintain reciprocal relationships, and the willingness to empower others (Goleman & Boyatzis, 2008). The most successful and productive healthcare teams are those in which the concept of the collective as leader is applied. This means that all members, regardless of status, are self-aware and committed to assuming leadership and responsibility for the continued development of the group.

This text is designed to help all health professionals realize their capacity for leadership and develop the knowledge, skills, and attitudes that are requisite to becoming a positive agent of change and growth in themselves, others, and their organizations.

This text is comprised of three parts: Teamwork and Group Development, Relationship-Centered Leadership, and Building and Sustaining Collaborative Interprofessional Teams. Each part is divided into chapters that introduce theoretical concepts, provide case stories, and active teaching/learning experiences that are appropriate for in-class, online, or personal reflective learning environments.

Part I: Teamwork and Group Development introduces groups as complex systems and includes models of group dynamics, the developmental stages of groups, and how to optimize teamwork throughout the group life span. Activities provide practice in differentiating personal from group goals, analyzing the developmental levels of groups, and applying strategies that individual leaders/members can employ to foster and sustain highly functional teams.

Part II: Relationship-Centered Leadership provides a detailed discussion of leadership behaviors, emotional intelligence, and how self-awareness, self-management, and an understanding of positive psychology can facilitate team development and productivity. Activities will help the reader analyze competencies required for health professions leadership; analyze leadership behaviors in real-life situations; identify personal leadership characteristics, challenges, philosophy, and behaviors; and conceptualize strategies for successful personal and health professional leadership for members as well as leaders of healthcare teams.

Part III: Building and Sustaining Collaborative Interprofessional Teams focuses on spanning professional boundaries, facilitating the development of a team culture, and generative practice. Practices that include appreciative inquiry and positive communication can facilitate the development of affiliative environments and help sustain the productivity and effectiveness of relationship-centered healthcare teams. Real-world profiles provide examples of these concepts in action. Activities will focus on helping the student develop interpersonal sensitivity and attentiveness, utilize empathic communication strategies, provide and receive feedback, use positive influence to build trust, manage conflict, and leverage the creativity and energy inherent to diverse healthcare teams.

References

Bray, M., Adamson, B., & Mason, M. (Eds.). (2007). *Comparative education research: Approaches and methods.* Hong Kong, China: Comparative Education Research Centre.

Brown, T. (2012). The boy who wanted to fly. *New York Times*, July 15, 2012.

Calhoun, J., Dollett, L., Sinioris, M., Wainio, J., Butler, P. Griffith, J., Warden, & G. (2008). Development of an interprofessional competency model for healthcare leadership. *Journal of Healthcare Management, 53*(6), 360–374.

Drinka, T., & Clark, P. (2000). *Health care teamwork: Interdisciplinary practice and teaching.* Westport, CT: Auburn House.

Dowd, M. (2012). Don't get sick in July. *New York Times*, July 15, 2012.

Frenk, J., Chen, L. Bhutta, Z., Cohen, J., Crisp, N., & Zurayk, H. (2010). Health professionals for a new century: Transforming education to strengthen health systems in an interdependent world. doi:10.1016/S0140-6736(10)61854-5

Freshman, B., Rubino, L., & Chassiako, Y. (2010). *Collaboration across the disciplines in health care*. Boston: Jones & Bartlett.

Gittell, J. (2009). *High performance healthcare: Using the power of relationships to achieve quality, efficiency and resilience*. New York, NY: McGraw Hill.

García, L. M., & Roblin, N. P. (2008). Innovation, research and professional development in higher education: Learning from our own experience. *Teaching and Teacher Education, 24*(1), 104–116.

Gray, B. (2008). Enhancing transdisciplinary research through collaborative leadership. *Am J Prev Med*, 35(2S), s124–s132.

Goleman, D., & Boyatzis, R. (2008, September). Social intelligence and the biology of leadership. *Harvard Business Review*, 86(9), 74–81.

Grant, R. W., & Finocchio, L. J., California Primary Care Consortium Subcommittee on Interdisciplinary Collaboration. (1995). *Interdisciplinary collaborative teams in primary care: A model curriculum and resource guide*. San Francisco, CA: Pew Health Professions Commission.

Institutes of Medicine. (1999). *To err is human: building a safer health system*. Washington, DC: Institutes of Medicine.

Institutes of Medicine. (2001). *Crossing the quality chasm: A new health system for the 21st century*. Washington, DC: National Academy Press.

Institutes of Medicine. (2002). *Who will keep the public healthy? Educating public health professionals for the 21st century*. Washington, DC: National Academy Press.

Institutes of Medicine. (2003). *Health professions education: A bridge to quality*. Washington, DC: National Academy Press.

Interprofessional Education Collaborative Expert Panel. (2011). *Core competencies for interprofessional collaborative practice: Report of an expert panel*. Washington, DC: Interprofessional Education Collaborative.

Hammick, M., Freeth, D., Copperman, J., & Goodsman, D. (2009). *Being interprofessional*. Malden, MA: Polity Press.

Lee, T. (2010). Turning doctors into leaders. *Harvard Business Review*, pp. 50–58.

Palincsar, A. (2007). Reflections on the special issue. *Educational Psychology Review, 19*(1), 85–89.

Pew Health Professions Commission. (1998). *Recreating health professional practice for a new century: The fourth report of the Pew Health Professions Commission.* San Francisco, CA: Pew Health Professions Commission.

Rowe, J. (2003). Approaching interdisciplinary research. In F. Kessel, P. Rosenfield, & N. Anderson (Eds.), *Expanding the boundaries of health and social science: Case studies in interdisciplinary innovation* (pp. 3–9). New York, NY: Oxford University Press.

Royeen, C., Jensen, G., & Harvan, R. (2009). *Leadership in Interdisciplinary Health Care Education and Practice.* Jones & Bartlett, Sudbury, MA.

Suchman, A., Sluyter, D., & Williamson, P. (2011). *Leading change in healthcare: Transforming organizations using complexity, positive psychology and relationship-centered care.* London, England: Radcliffe Publishing.

Wheelan, S. A., Burchill, C. N., & Tilin, F. (2003). The link between teamwork and patients' outcomes in intensive care units. *American Journal of Critical Care, 12*, 527–534.

World Health Organization: Health Professions Network Nursing and Midwifery Office within the Department of Human Resources for Health. (2010). *Framework for Action on Interprofessional Education & Collaborative Practice* (WHO/HRH/HPN/10.3). Geneva, Switzerland: World Health Organization. http://www.who.int/hrh/nursing_midwifery/en/

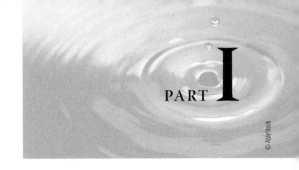

© AbleStock

Teamwork and Group Development

"When sufficient numbers of organization members become more self-aware, more concerned about the needs of others and more effective as group members and group leader—they cannot help but eventually have a positive influence on the total function and structure of any system."

Shaffer & Gallinsky, 1989, p. 192

Chapter 1: Groups-Teams-Systems

Chapter 2: Group Development

Chapter 3: Team Building Blocks

Part I Activities

Groups-Teams-Systems

Learning Objectives

1. Understand groups as complex, open systems.
2. Apply the concept of open systems to healthcare teams.
3. Differentiate groups and teams.
4. Describe levels of systems and how they relate to healthcare teams.
5. Understand how the diversity inherent to interprofessional healthcare teams contributes to their adaptability and sustainability.

Why Groups?

Humans are wired to be interdependent. We bond together in families, in friendship groups, in sports, neighborhoods, in work groups, and recently in electronic social networks like Facebook. The world has become more complex, and the exponential growth of information that is required to solve problems is not the purview of a single person or a single profession. By recognizing our need to join with others to meet these challenges, we

3

have the opportunity for collective wisdom to emerge. Facilitate the creation of new connections and innovative strategies to ensure the health and stability of the world that we share (Briskin, Erickson, Ott, & Callanan, 2009). Groups that we often refer to as teams have been and will continue to be an essential part of our daily lives. Nowhere is the need for teamwork more relevant than in the healthcare arena.

Diagnosis and intervention require the efforts of a cadre of physician specialists, nurses, therapists, pharmacists, social services personnel, laboratory personnel, information managers, dietitians, transportation workers, home health aides, family caregivers, and patients. Quality health care that is accessible and cost effective requires that the boundaries between these stakeholders are made permeable through consistent collaboration (Grant & Finocchio, 1995). Skills in team building, team membership, and the understanding of group dynamics are foundational and indispensable for the next generation of healthcare leaders. Well-functioning healthcare teams are linked to good morale, reduced staff turnover, and positive patient outcomes (Gittell, 2009; Lawrence, 2002; Torrens, 2010; Woltmann et al., 2008).

CASE STORY: *The Importance of Interprofessional Teams*

Here, everything is a committee decision. You can have input from multiple perspectives such as nursing, social work, occupational therapy, physical therapy, dietary. Elder problems are highly complicated. Getting other perspectives is helpful. For example, let's say you can't transport Mrs. X into the center because she keeps hitting people and is not putting her seatbelt on. What do you do? You need to get different perspectives in order to make a decision. It is like that example of the blind men and the elephant. No single perspective will describe the elephant and there probably is not one single resolution. This requires that team members are confident in what they know, amenable to listen to someone else's ideas and willing to offer their own ideas.

—Karen J. Nichols, MD, Chief Medical Officer, LIFE (Living Independently for Elders) Practice, School of Nursing, University of Pennsylvania.

What Distinguishes a Group from a Random Collection of People?

There is a unique designation for each of the myriad groupings in the animal kingdom such as school (fish), troop (baboons), murder (crows), gam (whales), and group (humans). No matter what the species, the critical element that is common to all the groupings is that the individual members are interdependent. In the case of humans, "members are linked together in a web of interpersonal relationships. Thus, a group is defined as two or more individuals who are connected to one another by social relationships" (Forsyth, 2006, pp. 2–3). Alderfer (1977) expanded the definition of human groups to include how they are distinguished from and perceived by nonmembers and how they relate to other groups. For the purposes of this text, in order for a group to be distinguished from a random collection of people, its members must have common interests and goals and regular patterns of interaction, exert influence among the members, and work interdependently to achieve goals (Cartright & Zander, 1968; Lewin, 1948; Smith, 2008; Wheelan, 2004).

What Is the Difference Between a Team and a Group?

Team and *group* are often used interchangeably. However, making the distinction between these two terms can offer valuable insight into how groups work and can facilitate leadership and full participation in productive teams. The term *group* comes from the French word *groupe* and from the Italian *gruppo*, which was borrowed originally from prehistoric Germanic *kruppaz*, which is translated into a "round mass, lump" (http://www.wordorigins .org/word-origins.com). This is hardly what we think of when we talk about work teams today. The term *group* is defined by Merriam Webster (2011, group entry) as "A number of individuals assembled together or having some unifying relationship." The origin of *team* is defined as a group that engages in more focused intentional action. The word derives from the Middle English term *teme* and the Old English *tēon* which is to draw or pull (Merriam Webster, 2011). Katzenbach and Smith (1993) describe

REFLECTION: *Identification of Groups*

Rank in order the 10 descriptions below with No. 1 being the most group-like and No. 10 the least grouplike. Give reasons for your rankings.

_____ The spectators at a college football game

_____ Two strangers exchanging meaningful looks across a crowded bar

_____ A secretary conversing with the boss by telephone

_____ Five students at a university working together on a classroom assignment

_____ A mob of rioters burning stores in the inner city

_____ Thirteen inmates talking and lifting weights in a jail's exercise yard

_____ A committee deciding the best way to handle a production problem

_____ Six employees working on an assembly line

_____ An aggregate of individuals waiting in silence for a bus

_____ The Smith family of Richmond, Virginia (Mr. Smith, Mrs. Smith, and Jane Smith, their daughter)

a *team* as "a small number of people with complementary skills who are committed to a common purpose, set of performance goals, and approach for which they hold themselves mutually accountable" (pp. 112).

The difference between a group and a team can be described on a continuum (**Figure 1-1**). At one end, *group* refers to people with something in common and at the other end of the spectrum *team* refers to people who must work together to get to

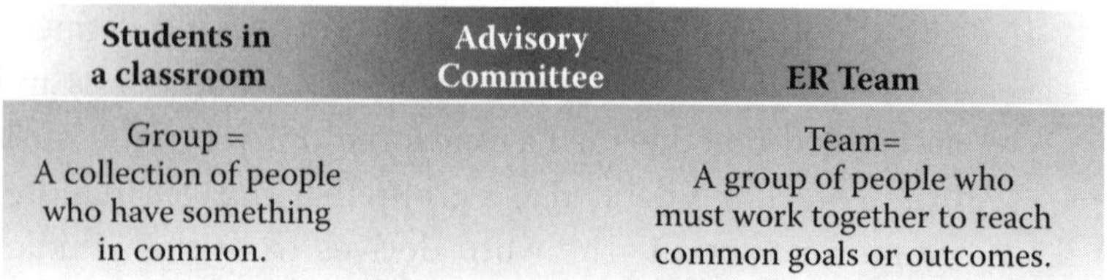

Students in a classroom	Advisory Committee	ER Team
Group = A collection of people who have something in common.		Team= A group of people who must work together to reach common goals or outcomes.

FIGURE 1-1 Group-team continuum.

a common agreed-upon goal or outcome. In this text, the term *group* will be used in discussions regarding the dynamics, processes, and patterns found in human collectives. Health professionals who are working together to achieve positive patient outcomes will be designated as *teams*.

A Systems Approach to Groups

Systems theory conceptualizes all physical and social systems as integrated wholes as opposed to agglomerations of disparate pieces. The eighteenth-century German philosopher, Hegel, introduced systems theory by suggesting that the whole is more than the sum of its parts, that the whole determines the nature of the parts, and the parts are dynamically interrelated and cannot be understood in isolation from the whole. The biologist Ludwig von Bertanffly proposed that all biological systems are open to each other and each identifiable component is related to other parts (Banathy, 1968). From a systems theory point of view, an individual member of a team cannot fully be understood in isolation from the team, and a team cannot be fully understood without understanding the organizational context within which it exists.

Katz and Kahn (1978) explored the open systems theory further when they proposed a method to analyze open (living) social systems using the systems theory. They posited that the interactive paradigm of analyzing living systems like organizations is based on continual cycles of input, throughput (processing), and outputs. All living organisms, like healthcare organizations and the groups that comprise them, are fully open systems. There are some key characteristics of open systems that resonate in the healthcare arena. Information from the external environment or input is provided by hospital staff, care recipients, suppliers, and funding sources. Intervention from health professionals is an example of throughput, while patient outcomes, patient satisfaction rates, and quality improvement outcomes are examples of system outputs (Meyer & O'Brien-Pallas, 2010).

Suchman, Sluyter, and Williamson (2011) provide an apt metaphor for healthcare organizations that is in keeping with the principles of open systems:

We can perceive a healthcare organization as a gigantic complicated conversation involving its staff, patients (and their families), payers, regulators, neighbors, competitors, and anyone else who interacts with or is affected by it. Within this gigantic conversation, there are . . . myriad [simultaneous] sub conversations . . . board meetings. . . . chance conversations at the water cooler . . . face to face or in virtual space . . . in the language of spoken or written words or of symbolic gestures . . . between individuals or in the private space of each person's thinking . . . Thinking of an organization as a conversation rather than a machine . . . [we] understand that we can influence but not control what goes on, and that we do so more by the way in which we participate than by the plans we make. (p. 15–16)

Each participant in a team takes in the ideas and opinions of others (input), processes this input and compares and integrates it with their most current thoughts (throughput), and together with the group, creates a new, collective perspective (output).

The organizational conversations reflect the organization's values, mission, culture, knowledge base, and interactive patterns or group dynamics. Organizations that attempt to impose a mechanistic, linear orientation upon an inherently open system such as a group, organization or community discount the value and challenges of randomness. These tightly coupled systems find themselves too rigid to respond to internal or external signals for the need to change. Change in open systems is inevitable, and adapting to these environmental changes is a continuous process. The manner in which groups and their parent organizations respond to change sets the boundaries for their collective creativity, productivity, and outcomes (Vickers, 1983; Weick, 1976).

Systems, subsystems, and the environment, while defined by boundaries, are interactive and interdependent. The dynamic relationship between structure and function of all aspects of the system and its environment render the boundaries permeable. Changes at any level of a system affect all other levels of the system.

For instance, organizational culture is as much a product of individual behaviors as it is a facilitator of individual behaviors

CONVERSATION DYNAMIC

Conversations allow us to inquire, exchange and process information, expand thinking, and negotiate and transform that information into a common perspective that is different than the sum of its parts.

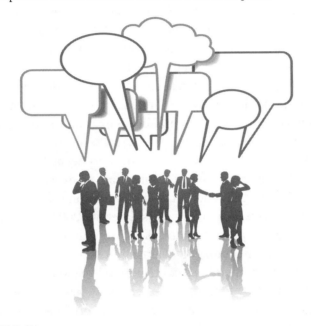

FIGURE 1-2

© Michael D Brown/ShutterStock, Inc.

(Studer, 2003). The mood of an individual leader can impact the mood of the team and be impacted by the tone of the team, or a team's effectiveness or ineffectiveness can impact and be impacted by the success of an organization. Nembhard & Edmondson (2006) found that inclusive behavior on the part of physician leaders yielded higher perceptions of psychological safety, increased engagement in all members of the healthcare team, and concomitant positive quality improvement efforts. Healthcare organizations that have been able to institutionalize relationship building as a means for integrating myriad systems consistently report higher staff retention rates and better clinical outcomes (Gittel, 2009; Singh, 2000; Woltmann et al., 2008).

Within all living systems, the balance between energy consumption (entropy) and energy infusion (negentropy) is necessary for the maintenance of a steady state for optimal systems functioning (homeostasis). An example of this in healthcare practice is the effect of caretaker rest (energy infusion) on patient care (indicates status of system's functioning). The relationship between decreased caretaker rest and decreased cognitive and clinical performance on the part of the caretaker and concomitant medical errors has been well documented (Reed, Fletcher, & Arora, 2010).

The evolutionary capacity of a system depends on flexible and adaptable patterns of organization that facilitate its ability to deal with environmental challenges and opportunities. The most agile, adaptable, and successful healthcare teams are those that are able to routinely evaluate who needs to be present and who has the most cogent information or expertise. Diverse perspectives and a broad range of information is essential for sound clinical decision making (Briskin et al., 2009; Wheatley, 2005). Inclusionary practices such as incorporating caregivers and support personnel into the healthcare team and equal recognition of each team member's contribution broaden the perspective of the team. In addition, increased psychological safety and willingness of members to share information facilitates the generation of innovative solutions for improved patient care (Meyer & O'Brien-Pallas, 2010; Nembhard & Edmondson, 2006).

Applying Systems Theory

When attempting to study, understand, and effect change in a social system, it is helpful to understand that there are levels of the system, which include individual, interpersonal, group, organizational, and community.

Individual: One person.
Interpersonal: Dyads.
Group: Three or more individuals working toward a common goal or purpose.
Organization: A social structure, often made up of groups, that pursues a collective goal to deliver some product or service.

Community: Anything beyond the organizational level. This includes other organizations, governments, or global social networks.

Systematic analysis and intervention is often targeted at the level of system where the impact will be the greatest. Successful change agents, whether they are leaders or members of groups, learn to differentiate between system levels and to shift attention from one level to another and make an informed decision about the best level at which to intervene based on a realistic appraisal of the change agent's sphere of influence (Gillette & McCollom, 1990; Wells, 1995). While the primary focus of this text is the group level of system, individual and interpersonal levels will also be explored. **Table 1-1** shows group-level intervention in relation to the other levels of system.

TABLE 1-1   Intervention at Each Level of System

Level	Focus	Goal	Methods
Individual	Individual's behavior, perceptions, and emotions.	Increase self-awareness and self-management.	Coaching, training, mentoring, and feedback.
Interpersonal	The relationship and communication between two people.	Clarify the nature of the relationship and goals and strengthen foundations for clear communication.	Conflict management, mediation, communication, and conflict resolution training.
Group	Group goals, tasks, roles.	Clarify the nature of individual contributions, the group's purpose, and group behaviors that will foster accomplishment of goals.	Education and feedback on the stages of group development, team building, leadership, and coaching behaviors that contribute to team effectiveness and productivity.

(continues)

TABLE 1-1 Intervention at Each Level of System *(Continued)*

Level	Focus	Goal	Methods
Organization	Culture, leadership development, and organizational strategy and structure.	Increase awareness of the people in the organization that the whole is different from the sum of its parts. Identify what attributes, behaviors, and strategies are necessary in order to reach the organizational goals.	Analysis of organizational state including culture, training in culture change, top team development, and executive coaching. Identify organizational strengths in order to leverage culture change, appreciative inquiry, and dynamic inquiry.
Community	Finding common ground so that the community can be served.	Building partnerships and collaborations across communities to deliver services.	Strategic planning, community development, and futuring.

LEVEL OF SYSTEMS CASE STUDY: *Stephanie's Dilemma*

The vice president of hospital facility services, Stephanie Scardola, was struggling with a problem.

A new human resources (HR) director for facilities services, Colin Doyle, was hired six months previously. In the past, this position was filled by former administrative assistants in the hospital system and served as a professional development step towards a more responsible management positions. Most of the people who held this position left within two years to go on to another position in the hospital or in another hospital system. The committee felt that it was time to hire someone with more HR experience and with an outsider's point of view even though the compensation and job level was still the same.

Colin came from a small, nonprofit company and has eight years of HR experience. He never worked in a hospital nor did he have union experience; however, the committee hired him because he was the most experienced candidate, had a master's degree in HR, and was professional and knowledgeable. This HR position reports to both the vice president of facility services and an HR director from the hospital's central HR department. The duties include partnering with managers in the facilities department, helping them deal with union and nonunion discipline issues, being responsible for getting people paid properly, and making sure all of the proper paperwork is in order and sent to central HR.

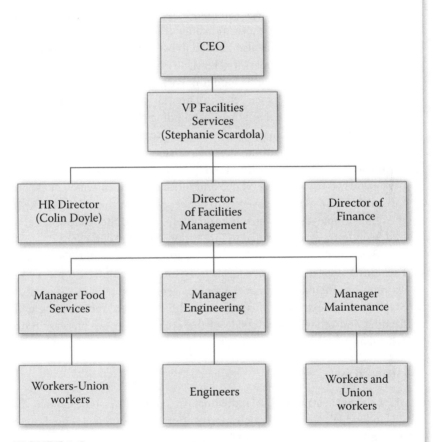

FIGURE 1-3

When Colin was first hired, he performed well. He conducted several employee orientation training sessions and was able to put two new policies in place to assist the facilities services managers in handling some situations on their own. Unfortunately, problems began a few months later. Colin was not keeping up with emails, he made some vital mistakes with

(continues)

some employees under union contracts, and he overpaid two employees, along with other issues.

Stephanie met with Colin about all of these issues and each time there were valid reasons why errors occurred. He informed Stephanie that employees often took issues directly to central HR, bypassing him, and therefore he did not know about those problems until it was too late to solve them. Managers were either not coming to him with issues or also were coming after the damage was already done. He did remind Stephanie that he was on a learning curve and some of the mistakes were due to his own lack of experience. He also needed to become more familiar with the new union contract. On a personal level, he said there was too much on his plate; he was a single dad and could not work late every night.

About three months earlier, the Director of Facilities Management left his position and Stephanie had been filling this role as well as taking care of her duties as a member of the senior team of the hospital. Due to this position, she was getting direct feedback from managers that Colin did not answer his emails. Although he was responsive when addressed in person, he was sometimes a bit glib and rule based and answered questions too quickly. The managers were also concerned that when Colin spoke to the union employees he was too sympathetic toward them. He seemed to buddy up to them and seemed to lose his professional demeanor.

The Chief Executive Officer (CEO) found out that the Director of Facilities Management position was open and would remain that way for six months. The managers, at this point, were all reporting to Stephanie. Stephanie was extremely busy running the operation and working with funding and other issues outside of the organization, which were more critical parts of her responsibilities.

QUESTIONS:

1. Look at the row labeled "Individual" in Table 1.1. Assume Colin is the individual. Describe which intervention technique you would apply and how this would positively impact Colin's behavior.

2. Look at the row labeled "group" in Table 1.1. Assume the group consists of Stephanie and the three Directors. Describe which intervention technique you would apply and how this could help this group better reach its goals.

3. You are the CEO. Look at the row labeled "organization" in Table 1.1. Describe which intervention technique you would apply and how this could make a positive impact on Stephanie's Dilemma.

4. After looking at this from all three perspectives, what do you think would be the preferred way to handle the issue?

References

Alderfer, C. P. (1977). Organization development. *Annual Review of Psychology, 28*, 197–223.

Banathy, B. H., & Jenlink, P. M. (2004). Systems inquiry and its application in education. In D. H. Jonassen (Ed.) *Handbook of Research on Educational Communications and Technology* (p. 37–57). Mahwah, NJ.: Lawrence Erlbaum Associates

Briskin, A., Erickson, S., Ott, J., & Callanan, T. (2009). *The power of collective wisdom and the trap of collective folly*. San Francisco, CA: Berrett-Koehler.

Cartright, D., & Zander, A. (1968). *Group dynamics: Research and theory*, New York, NY: Harper & Row Publishers.

Forsyth, D. R. (2006). *Group dynamics* (4th ed. [international student ed.]). Belmont CA: Thomson Wadsworth Publishing.

Gillette & McCollom, M. (1990). *Groups in context: A new perspective on group dynamics*: Lanham, MD: University Press.

Gittell, J. (2009). *High performance healthcare: Using the power of relationships to achieve quality, efficiency and resilience*. New York, NY: McGraw-Hill.

Grant R., & Finocchio, L., California Primary Care Consortium Subcommittee on Interdisciplinary Collaboration. (1995). *Interdisciplinary collaborative teams in primary care: A model curriculum and resource guide*. San Francisco, CA: Pew Health Professions Commission.

Group. (2011). In *Merriam-Webster.com*. Retrieved from http://www.merriam-webster.com/dictionary/group

Katz, D. & Kahn,R. (1978). *The social psychology of organizations*. Hoboken, NJ: Wiley.

Katzenbach, J.R. & Smith, D.K. (1993). *The Wisdom of Teams: Creating the High-performance Organization*. Boston: Harvard Business School.

Lawrence, D. (2002). *From chaos to care: The promise of team based medicine*. Cambridge, MA: Perseus Publishing.

Lewin, K. (1948). *Resolving social conflicts: Selected papers on group dynamics*. Gertrude W. Lewin (Ed.). New York, NY: Harper & Row.

Meyer, R. M., & O'Brien-Pallas, L. L. (2010). Nursing services delivery theory: An open system approach. *Journal of Advanced Nursing, 66*(12), 2828–2838.

Nembhard, I., & Edmondson, A. (2006). Making it safe: The effects of leader inclusiveness and professional status on psychological safety and improvement efforts in health care teams. *Journal of Organizational Behavior, 27*, 941–966.

Reed, D., Fletcher, K., & Arora, V. (2010). Systemic review: Association of shift length, protected sleep time and night float with patient care, residents' health and education. *Annals of Internal Medicine, 153*, 829–842.

Singh, S. (2000). Running an effective community mental health team. *Advances in Psychiatric Treatment, 6*, 414–422.

Smith, M. (2008). *Experience in groups and other papers*. New York, NY: Tavistock Publications Limited.

Studer, Q. (2003). *Hardwiring excellence: Purpose, worthwhile work, making a difference*. Gulf Breeze, FL: Fire Starter Publishing.

Suchman, A., Sluyter, D., & Williamson, P. (2011). *Leading change in healthcare: Transforming organizations using complexity, positive psychology and relationship-centered care*. London, England: Radcliffe Publishing.

Team. (2011). In *Merriam-Webster.com*. Retrieved from http://www.merriam-webster.com/dictionary/team

Torrens, P. (2010). The health care team members: Who are they and what do they do? In F. Freshman, B. Rubino, & Chassiakos Y. (Eds.), *Collaboration across the disciplines in health care* (pp. 1–19). Sudbury, MA: Jones and Bartlett Learning.

Vickers, G. (1983). *Human systems are different*. London, England: Harper and Row.

Weick, K. (1976). Educational organizations as loosely coupled systems, *Administrative Science Quarterly, 21*, 1, 1–19.

Wells, L. (1995). The group as a whole: A systemic socio-analytic perspective on interpersonal and group relations. In G. Gillette, & M. McCollum (Eds.), *Groups in context* (pp. 50–85) Lanham, MD: University Press of America.

Wheatley, M. (2005). *Finding our way.* San Francisco, CA: Berret-Koehler Publishers, Inc.

Woltmann, E., Whitley, R., McHugo G., Brunette, M., Torrey, W. Coots, L., Drake, R. (2008, July). The role of staff turnover in the implementation of evidence-based practices in mental health care. *Psychiatric Services, 59*, 732–737.

CHAPTER 2

Group Development

Learning Objectives

1. Discuss aspects of small group behavior theory as described in the literature.
2. Systematically examine the conscious and unconscious components of group life.
3. Differentiate the developmental stages of group life.
4. Analyze group behavior.
5. Facilitate teamwork throughout the group life span.

The Group

As members or leaders of groups, most of us notice the personalities of the members of the group, the topics discussed, the disagreements, and our own emotions. While individualistic Western cultures routinely view groups as collections of individuals, Eastern cultures have long recognized groups as distinct collectives rather than a collection of distinct individuals (Hofstede, 1983).

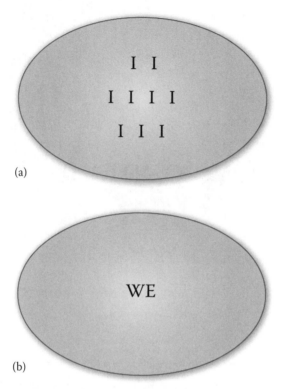

(a)

(b)

FIGURE 2-1 The *I*/*We* perception.

This perspective informs the way the group harnesses its power in order to get something done. Shifting from an *I* perspective to a *We* perspective recognizes the group as a source of intelligence that is greater than any one individual and facilitates the integration, engagement, and creation of collective wisdom—ultimately achieving a whole that is more powerful and creative than the sum of its parts (Briskin, Erickson, Ott, & Callanan, 2009).

All groups demonstrate consistent patterns of member, leader, and group behaviors as they relate to the acquisition of roles, the assumption of and response to authority, norm development, and communication patterns. These patterns serve as indicators of developmental changes in the group over time. Neuroscience supports the notion of a social brain—a neurophysiological conduit for perceiving, processing, and mirroring the emotions and behaviors of others. In other words, our interactions with each other in groups have the potential to trigger neuronal activity, which, in turn, influences our emotions and behaviors (Goleman, 2011). Positive or negative action on the part of one person can trigger a like reaction in another. When repeated often enough, this positive or negative interaction pattern becomes a group norm (Frederickson, 2003).

We have all experienced a time when we were in sync or on the same wavelength or connected with another individual or group of individuals on a level that transcended the social psychological aspects of engagement. Integrating the systemic laws of neuropsychology and physics with social psychology, Rene Levi (2005) examined and labeled these transcendent experiences as "collective resonance" and defined it as:

> A felt sense of energy, rhythm, or intuitive knowing that occurs in a group of human beings and positively affects the way they interact toward a positive purpose . . . that enables us to make greater progress toward our common human goals than we have been able to do using idea exchange and analytic problem-solving alone. (p. 1)

This view is consistent with the "*Weness*" inherent to the Eastern conceptualization of groups and the emergence of collective intelligence in collectives of all types—including teams, organizations, and communities. It is important to note that these potentially generative interactive and integrative tendencies that are inherent to humans—when not managed mindfully—can devolve into collective folly with a focus on the barriers that divide and polarize rather than the connections that unify (Briskin, 2009).

These interactive patterns, carried out over the life of the group, contribute to the development of a unique social organism that is more than the sum of its parts (Bion, 1974; Lewin, 1951; Perls, Hefferline, & Goodman, 1951; Tilin & Broder, 2005; Tuckman, 1965; Wheelan, 2005).

Each of the columns in **Table 2-1** represents a level of system in the group life—the group as a unit, the individual members within the group, and the context or the environment within which the group exists. Under each component are aspects that

TABLE 2-1

Member	Group	Environment
Behavior—How does each member behave in the group?	**Norms/rules**—What are the explicit/tacit rules for behavior in this group?	**Physical/social proximity**—How much time does the group spend together?
Personal feelings—How do each of the members feel about working in the group?	**Roles**—Who are the talkers/listeners?	**Relations with outsiders**—What is stronger—members' intragroup or extragroup relations?
Internalized norms—What are the personal rules that are held by each member?	**Authority**—Who are the leaders/followers?	**Responsibilities/ expectations**—What is expected of this group?
Beliefs/values—What beliefs/values influence each member?	**Communication**—Who talks to whom?	**Cultural issues**—What are the cultural issues (age, ethnic, gender, professional) that might impact this group?
Self-concept—How does each member see himself or herself functioning in the group?		**Level of autonomy**—How much control over the outcomes of this group does the group have?

contribute to the social–psychological landscape of every group at any point in time. The study of group dynamics attempts to analyze and interpret group life by examining these aspects in a systematic fashion.

What You See Is Not What You Get: The Unconscious Life of a Group

Wilfred Bion, a psychoanalyst, was one of the first researchers to identify patterns in groups. Bion maintained that groups have a conscious and an unconscious life. He named the conscious group the *work group* and the unconscious group the *basic assumption group.* The conscious work group focuses on rationally accomplishing overt tasks and activities. The basic assumption group describes the unconscious aspects of a group. Leaders and members often mistakenly perceive these unconscious aspects as interfering with the real work of the group. In fact, this is the way that the collective membership and leadership of the group deal with the anxiety and polarities of individual identity and collective identity. Bion specifically identified the following three basic assumptions: dependency, fight-flight, and pairing (see **Table 2-2**). Leaders and members who learn to identify these group processes as a natural part of a group's development are better prepared to be positive catalysts in the group. Rather than being caught up in the anxiety of the group, this knowledge can allow a person to be more objective, emotionally independent, and prepared to act in a constructive manner (Bennis & Shepherd, 1956, p. 417–418).

Stages of Group Development

While there are multiple factors that influence group functioning, each group—like each human being—should be considered a unique organism that passes through predictable phases of development. Characteristic member, leader, and group behaviors, as they relate to the acquisition of roles, the assumption of and response to authority, norm development, and communication patterns—like human developmental milestones—serve as indicators of developmental changes in the group over time. Awareness of the interacting determinants of group behavior and the unconscious assumptions of the group will facilitate an understanding of group behavior and facilitate effective group leadership and participation.

Groups display behavioral patterns that are common to all groups and are not dependent on the individuals in the group. A number of theorists have used various terms to describe the key issues that groups address over their life span. While these issues are ever present, some issues gain primacy depending upon the developmental level of the group. In summary, the group, as a

TABLE 2-2 Wilfred Bion Summary

		Group Aim	Anxiety	Member	Leader	Behavior
Unconscious	Dependency	Security	Anxiety is reduced through leader's superhuman ability to care for the group.	Knows nothing, inadequate and childlike.	Omnipotent, parent and protector.	Leader makes all decisions, provides all direction, and solves all problems.
	Fight or flight	Balance group identity with individual identities	Anxiety is expressed by resisting or fleeing the group dynamic.	Paradoxically struggles to balance group identity with personal identity.	Leader loses omnipotent status and is often blamed for not resolving the individual vs. group problem.	Fluctuates between arguing and avoiding difficult topics. Scapegoating: Individuals and leaders can be sacrificed for the sake of the group.
	Pairing	Hope and optimism	Anxiety is reduced by letting the pair take control.	Let the pair do the work.	The pair acts on behalf of a leader.	Two people in the group take on the task of working out the unconscious group dilemmas.
Conscious	Work group	Fulfills the actual goals and tasks of a group	Anxiety is reduced enough to focus on work.	Contributes to the group reaching its goals.	Contributes to the group reaching its goals.	Leaders and members will support the group to achieve tangible goals.

Data from: Bion, W (1974) *Experiences in Groups: And other papers.* Paolo Alto, CA: Science and Behavior Books, Inc.

whole, struggles to find the right balance between the unconscious desire to have a group identity and retain individual identities. Over time, a group is also challenged with dealing with the paradox of being safely protected by an omnipotent leader and taking control of its own destiny. A mature group learns to deal effectively with these issues. Its members work cooperatively as separate and discrete members who willingly choose to belong to the group because they identify with interests of the group. This group tests its conclusions, seeks knowledge, learns from its experience, and is in agreement with regard to the group's purpose and tasks (Bales, 1950; Bion, 1974; Rioch, 1983; Schutz, 1958; Tuckman, 1965; Wheelan, 2005; Yalom, 1995).

Tuckman (1965) conducted an extensive review of the group development literature and concluded that therapy groups, work groups, and human relations training groups (t-groups)[1] had strong developmental similarities despite differences in group composition, task, goal, and the duration of group life. He noted a few critical common themes about groups:

1. There is a distinction between groups as a social entity and a task entity.
2. In all groups, the task and the social emotional functions occur simultaneously.
3. All groups go through four stages of group development. The task and social emotional functions are different for each stage.
4. The group moves from one stage to the next by successfully accomplishing the task and social emotional/group structure function at each stage.

Tuckman named these stages of group development *forming*, *storming*, *norming*, and *performing* (**Table 2-3**). He later added a fifth stage called *adjourning*, which describes the characteristics of groups as they terminate.

---

[1] Work groups and t-groups were categorized together in this literature review because there were not many natural studies of workplace groups at the time.

TABLE 2-3 Tuckman's Description of the Stages of Group Development Based on Literature Review of Therapy and T-Groups

Tuckman (1965)	Task Issues	Structure and Social-Emotional Issues
Forming	**Orientation to the task:** Group members attempt to define the group task by identifying information that will be needed and the ground rules that must be followed to complete the job of the group.	**Testing and dependence:** Group members attempt to discover acceptable behavior according to the leader and other group members.
Storming	**Emotional response to task demands:** Group members act emotionally to task demands and exhibit resistance to suggested actions.	**Intragroup conflict:** Group members disagree with one another and the leader as a way to express their own individuality.
Norming	**Discussing oneself and others:** Group members listen to each other and the leader and use information and input from everyone.	**Development of group cohesion:** Group members accept the group and the individuality of fellow members, thus becoming an entity through rule agreement and role clarification.
Performing	**Emergence of insight:** A variety of methods of inquiry are used and members adjust their behavior to serve the greater goals of the group.	**Functional role relatedness:** Members are focused on getting the task done and relate to each other in ways that will accomplish the task.

Data from: Tuckman, B. (1965). "Developmental Sequence in Small Groups." *Psychological Bulletin, 63*(6), 384–394.

An Integrated Model of Group Development

Susan Wheelan (2005) used empirical research to build on Tuckman's model. She proposed and validated an integrated model of group development using the Group Development Questionnaire (GDQ) (Wheelan, 1990; Wheelan & Hochberger, 1996). Using observational and survey data, this integrated model is consistent with previous models in that it describes group stages developing naturally and in a chronological fashion over time. In addition, Wheelan and her team of researchers found that:

- There are specific characteristics that emerge in each stage of a group's development. Early stages of group development are associated with specific issues and patterns of speech such as those related to dependency, counter dependency, and trust, which precede the actual work conducted during the more mature stages of a group's life.
- Groups navigate through the stages by accomplishing process-oriented goals like achieving a certain degree of member safety, expressing and tolerating different opinions, and devising agreed-upon methods of decision making.
- There is a normative time frame that most groups need in order to traverse each stage.
- Organizational culture influences group norms and can influence group development.
- Member and leader behaviors are equally important in the development of a group and the dynamic between them must be addressed as the group develops.

Identifying the Stages of Group Development: Characteristics and Goals

While stages of group development are identified by the issues that predominate, there is always a percentage of group energy that is expended on dependency, conflict, trust and work regardless of the stage. For example, work gets done at every stage of development. In earlier stages, most of the work is done under the leader's direction. In succeeding stages members take increasingly more responsibility. By Stages 3 and 4, responsibility for work is evenly distributed among the members and the leader is used as a resource. The key challenge for group members and leaders is finding the balance between task and social-emotional issues and managing the conflict that these issues engender over the life span of the group. Wheelan and Williams (2003) found that the communication content of groups over their life span mirror key

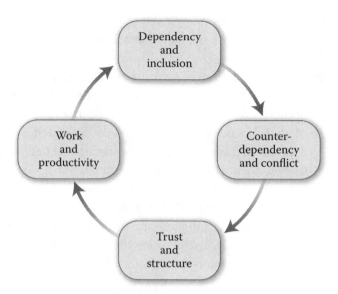

FIGURE 2-2 Key developmental issues of group life.

Data from: Wheelan, S. (2005). *Group Processes: A developmental perspective.* Boston: Allyn and Bacon.

developmental issues. In other words, the amount of time spent talking about task related concerns increases over the life of the group while the amount of time talking about social-emotional concerns decreases as the group matures. Figures 2-3A, B, and C provide an example of how the proportion of attention on key issues might shift based on the developmental level of the group. As with people, no one size fits all and each group ultimately demonstrates unique developmental patterns.

Stage I (Dependency/Inclusion) is characterized by significant member dependency on the designated leader, concerns about safety, and inclusion issues. In this stage, members rely on the leader and powerful group members to provide direction. This is manifested by the percentage of statements that address dependency and pairing (when two people couple or pair by giving mutual compliments to each other) (8% and 16%, respectively). Statements regarding conflict are few (about 6%). About 17% of the time, team members engage in safe, non controversial discussions filled with flight statements by exchanging stories about

Stage I

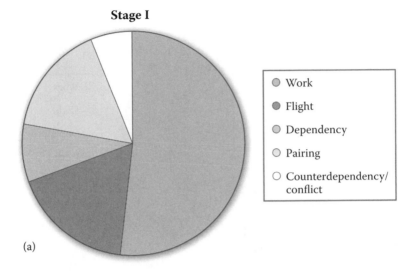

(a)

FIGURE 2-3A

Data from: Wheelan, S. (2005). *Group Processes: A developmental perspective.* Boston: Allyn and Bacon.

outside activities or other topics that are not relevant to group goals while approximately 50% of the time is spent on work related issues. The goals at Stage I are to: create a sense of belonging and the beginnings of predictable patterns of interaction, develop member loyalty to the group, and create an environment in which members feel safe enough to contribute ideas and suggestions.

Stage II (Counterdependency/Fight) is characterized by member disagreement about group goals and procedures and conflict is an inevitable. Flight statements decrease to about 7% and work statements remain at 49%. Dependency statements fall to 2% and those regarding conflict rise to 28%. Expressing disagreements and working them out is a necessary part of this process and allows members to communicate and begin to establish a trusting climate in which members feel free to disagree with each other and collaborate. The goals for Stage 2 are to: develop a unified set of goals, values, and operational procedures, and to strike a balance between respect for the individual contributions and mediating individual needs with the group needs.

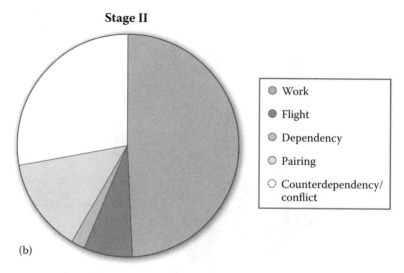

(b)

FIGURE 2-3B

Data from: Wheelan, S. (2005). *Group Processes: A developmental perspective.* Boston: Allyn and Bacon.

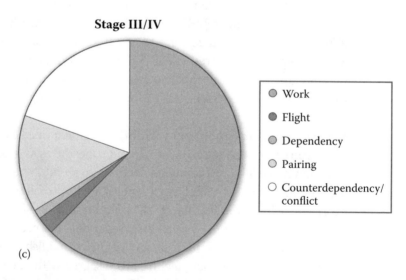

(c)

FIGURE 2-3C

Data from: Wheelan, S. (2005). *Group Processes: A developmental perspective.* Boston: Allyn and Bacon.

Stage III (Trust/Structure) is characterized by more mature negotiations about roles, organization, and procedures. The primary goal for Stage III is to solidify positive relationships that benefit the productivity of the group.

Stage IV (Work/Productivity) is characterized by a time of intense team productivity and effectiveness. Having resolved many of the issues of the previous stages, the group can focus most of its energy on goal achievement and task accomplishment.

TABLE 2-4 Wheelan: An Integrated Model of Group Development

Stage	Members	Group	Leader
I: Dependency/ Inclusion	• Tentative and polite • High compliance • Rarely express disagreement • Fear rejection • Conflict limited • Conformity high	• Assumes consensus • Roles based on external status and first impressions • Communication centralized • Lacks structure and organization	• Seen as benevolent and competent • Is expected to provided direction and safety • Is rarely challenged • Leader should facilitate communications safety & set standards
II: Counter dependency/ Fight	• Disagree about goals and tasks • Feel safer to dissent • Challenge the leader • Increase participation	• Conflicts emerge • Goal and role clarification begins • Decreasing conformity • Subgroups form • Intolerance for subgroups • Conflict management attempted • Successful conflict resolution increases consensus (i.e., goals) and culture • Trust and cohesion increases	• Is challenged frequently • Leader should help develop values, accept changes, and encourage independence.

TABLE 2-4   Wheelan: An Integrated Model of Group Development
(Continued)

Stage	Members	Group	Leader
III: Trust/ Structure	• Satisfaction increases • Commitment to group tasks is high	• Increased goal clarity and consensus • Communications structure more flexible • Communications content more task oriented	• Becomes less directive and more consultative • Leaders should be less directive, egalitarian, and more consultative
IV: Work/ Productivity	• Clear about group goals • Agree with group goals • Clear about their roles • Voluntary conformity is high • Cooperative	• Role assignments match member abilities • Communications structure matches task demands • Open communication allows participation of all members • Receives, gives, and uses feedback • Plans how to solve problems and make decisions • Implements and evaluates solutions and decisions • Highly cohesive • Task-related deviances tolerated	Style matches group developmental level Delegates Leaders should move toward non-leadership

Data from: Wheelan, S. (2005). *Group Processes: A developmental perspective.* Boston: Allyn and Bacon.

Roughly 62% of statements are related to work and 20% of the time is spent on sorting out differences of opinion on how the work should get done. At this point the group is resilient enough to remain cohesive while encouraging task-related conflicts.

REFLECTION: *Identify the Stage of a Group*

Which stage does the behavior indicate?

- Members are listening and seeking to understand one another.
- Members attempt to figure out their roles and functions.
- Divisive feelings and subgroups within the group increase.
- Group members follow a self-appointed or designated leader's suggestions without enthusiasm.
- Disagreements become more civilized and less angry and emotional.
- Members argue with one another, even when they agree on the basic issues.

Termination: When groups face their own ending point, some may address separation issues and members' appreciation of each other and the group experience. In other groups the impending end may cause disruption and conflict.

How Does the Stage of the Group Impact Team Productivity?

Wheelan (2005) found that aspects such as group size and group age affect development and productivity. It usually takes at least six months for a group to achieve the Stage IV developmental level. Newly formed groups are characterized by a higher percentage of dependency counterdependency/flight statements ("I don't know what to do." "The leader is incompetent." "Did you see the game last night?"), while more established groups make more work statements ("Let's focus on the task at hand."). These findings are corroborated by Nembhard & Edmondson (2006), who found that long-standing membership in healthcare teams was correlated with the willingness of all members, irrespective of status, to share information and provide innovative solutions— behaviors that are indicative of more mature groups.

In a study involving 17 intensive care units, Wheelan, Davidson, and Tilin (2003) found a link between perceived group maturity and patients' outcomes in intensive care units. Staff members of units with mortality rates that were lower than predicted perceived their teams as functioning at higher stages of group development. They perceived their team members as less dependent and more trusting than did staff members of units with mortality rates that were higher than predicted. Staff members of high-performing units also perceived their teams as more structured and organized than did staff members of lower performing units.

Group Size: Less Is More

It is not uncommon to hear members of groups complain that some members of the group are doing more work than others. This perceptual phenomenon can happen in any sized group but studies show that the larger the group, the less energy any individual exerts. In the late nineteenth century, Maximillian Ringelman performed one of the first experiments with group size by having groups of people pulling on a rope. He discovered that the more people pulled on a rope, the less each individual contributed. Ringelman called this phenomenon "social loafing." In

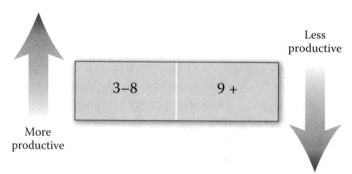

FIGURE 2-4 Correlation of group size and productivity. According to Wheelan, groups of three to eight were more productive and more mature at six months than groups with nine or more members.

Data from: Wheelan, S.A. (2009). Group size, group development, and productivity. *Small Group Research, 40*(2), 247–262

addition, larger groups tend to have a more difficult time coalescing around a single identity and distributing work in an equitable fashion. Studies indicate that cohesion and intimacy decrease as team size increases (Bogart & Lundgren, 1974; Fisher, 1953; Seashore, 1954). Members of larger groups perceive their groups to be more competitive, less cohesive, more argumentative and less satisfying (Steiner, 1972). Wheelan (2009) found that small groups tended to be more productive than large groups and small groups reached mature levels of group development more rapidly than large groups.

The literature seems to indicate that groups are most productive when they are composed of five to eight members. Theoretically, this is because the larger the group, the longer and more difficult it is for the group to develop a common identity.

CASE STORY: *How Many People are Needed to Make this Decision?*

Our team needs to make decisions regarding who should be enrolled in the program. There are applications that could potentially be denied for various reasons. When I first got here, there were 40 people in the morning meeting where these decisions were made. Everyone read the report at that meeting and, after the coffee kicked in, people were talking amongst themselves, others were listening, and others were on cell phones. People were just getting confused and the decision process was taking around two hours. I worked with the marketing people and changed this system. We now have a separate smaller group of 8 people in a meeting that includes social work, nursing, a physician, transportation and four marketing people who give input but don't get a vote. We invite additional guests from other departments such as behavioral medicine as needed.

At first, there was a lot of stress associated with the transition because change is stressful. But after six months the length of time from intake to decision was cut dramatically. The morning meeting can be done in 15 minutes!

—Karen J. Nichols, MD, Chief Medical Officer, University of Pennsylvania Life Program

How Long Does It Take for a Group to Develop Through Each Stage?

The most common question team leaders ask us is, "How can I get my team to develop faster?" If teams could develop faster, work productivity would go up, problems would be solved faster, and disagreements would easily be resolved. Research supports that it takes time for groups to mature (Wheelan, Davidson & Tilin, 2003). Under the right circumstances, groups can reach full maturity in six to eight months. Attempting to rush the process would be like expecting a 5-year-old child to behave like a 25-year-old adult. It would not yield good results and would only serve to frustrate everyone involved.

Figure 2-5 is meant to be a guide to the average amount of time researchers have ascribed to the stages of development based on the integrated model of group development. Every group is a bit different, and some may actually get stuck at a certain level of development and take longer to move on to the next stage. Issues such as culture, diversity, group management, organizational dynamics, and complexity of tasks, as well as group

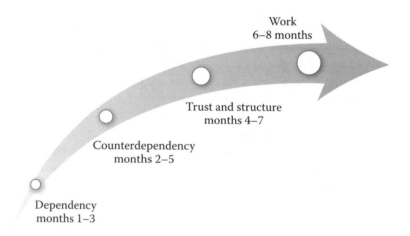

Work
6–8 months

Trust and structure
months 4–7

Counterdependency
months 2–5

Dependency
months 1–3

FIGURE 2-5 Time it takes for groups to mature.

Adapted from: Wheelan, S. Davidson, B., & Tilin, F. (2003). Group Development Across Time: Reality or Illusion? *Small Group Research, 34*(2), 223–245.

commitment and identity impact group dynamics and the way groups develop.

References

Bales, R. (1950). *Interaction process analysis: A method for the study of small groups.* Reading,MA: Addison-Wesley.

Bennis, W. G., & Shepherd, H. A. (1956). A theory of group development. *Human Relations, 9,* 415–437.

Bion, W. (1974). *Experiences in groups: And other papers.* Paolo Alto, CA: Science and Behavior Books, Inc.

Bogart, D., & Lundgren, D. (1974). Group size, member dissatisfaction, and group radicalism. *Human Relations, 27*(4), 339–355.

Briskin, A., Erickson, S., Ott, J., & Callanan, T. (2009). *The power of collective wisdom and the trap of collective folly.* San Francisco, CA: Berrett-Koehler.

Fisher, P. H. (1953). An analysis of the primary group. *Sociometry, 16,* 272–276.

Frederickson, B. (2003, July/August). The value of positive emotions. *American Scientist, 91,* 330–335.

Goleman, D. (2011). *Leadership: The power of emotional intelligence.* Northampton, MA: More Than Sound.

Hofstede, G. (1983). The cultural relativity of organizational practices and theories. *Journal of International Business Studies, 14*(2), 75–89.

Levi, R. (2005). What is resonance? Retrieved from http://resonanceproject.org/welcome1.cfm?pt=0&id=73

Nembhard, I., & Edmondson, A. (2006). Making it safe: The effects of leader inclusiveness and professional status on psychological safety and improvement efforts in health care teams. *Journal of Organizational Behavior, 27,* 941–966.

Perls, F., Hefferline, R., & Goodman, P. (1951). *Gestalt therapy: Excitement and growth in the human personality.* New York, NY: Julian Press.

Rioch, M,J. (1983). The work of Wilfred Bion in groups. In Coleman, A. & Bexron, W.H. (Ed). *Group relations reader 1* (pp. 21–32). Washington, D.D.: A.K. Rice Institute Series.

Schutz, W. (1958). *FIRO: A three dimensional theory of interpersonal behavior.* New York, NY: Rinehart.

Seashore, S. (1954). *Group cohesiveness in the industrial work group.* Ann Arbor, MI: Institute for Social Research.

Steiner, I. (1972). Group process and productivity. New York, NY: Academic Press.

Tilin, F., & Broder, J. (2005). Team consultation. In S. A. Wheelan (Ed.), *The handbook of group research and practice* (pp. 427–439). Thousand Oaks, CA: Sage Publications.

Tuckman, B. (1965). Developmental sequence in small groups. *Psychological Bulletin, 63*(6), 384–394.

Wheelan, S. (1990). Facilitating training groups: A guide to leadership and verbal intervention skills. New York, NY: Praeger.

Wheelan S. (2005) *Group Process: A developmental perspective, 2nd edition.* Needham Heights, MA: Allyn & Bacon.

Wheelan, S. A. (2009). Group size, group development, and productivity. *Small Group Research, 40*(2), 247–262.

Wheelan, S., Davidson, B., & Tilin, F. (2003). Group development across time: Reality or illusion? *Small Group Research, 34*(2), 223–245.

Wheelan, S., & Hochberger, J. (1996). Validation studies of the group development questionnaire. *Small Group Research, 27*(1), 143–170.

Yalom, I. (1995). *The theory and practice of group psychotherapy (4th edition).* New York: Basic Books.

CHAPTER 3

Team Building Blocks: Norms, Goals, Roles, Communication, Leaders, and Members

© AbleStock

Learning Objectives

1. Analyze how personal values and other motivating forces influence group process and development.
2. Differentiate personal and group needs.
3. Analyze the relationship between role assumption, group needs, and goal attainment.
4. Understand the relationship between communication and learning styles.
5. Match communication style to the needs of the listener.
6. Give and receive feedback.

Norms

Group norms are agreed-upon standards of behavior. Norms are the shared explicit or implicit rules that a group uses to identify standards of performance and distinguish appropriate from

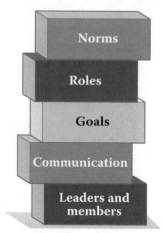

FIGURE 3-1

inappropriate behavior. When group norms are explicit or made explicit, they are commonly referred to as ground rules, agreements, group charters, conditions, or guidelines. However, not all norms are explicit, and the perceptions and concomitant behavior of individuals in groups is profoundly—and often unconsciously—affected by social influence (Sherif, 1936).

In many progressive organizations, errors are routinely considered teaching moments that can provide opportunities for open discussion, team-based problem solving and continuous organizational improvement. While similar normative responses to errors would elicit the same type of team and organization improvements in health care, the dire consequences of medical mistakes tend to discourage the very discussions that are necessary to prevent their occurrence (O'Daniel & Rosenstein, 2008). This tendency, in combination with differing professional identities, cultures, skills, domains of concern, differences in power, capacity, resources, goals, and accountability actually requires that more attention be paid to constructing organization-wide standards that encourage and reward interaction. In groups where intraprofessional and interprofessional conflict avoidance is the normative behavior, the ensuing misunderstandings and related mistrust tend to limit collaborative or cooperative behavior. Sustainable collaborative environments for interprofessional healthcare teams require a collectively constructed core of prescriptive

> **REFLECTION:** *Explicit and Implicit Norms in a Group*
>
> Identify the norms or rules of your work group.
>
> Interview members of your group and ask them to identify the rules of your group.
>
> How does your response differ from your coworkers? How is it the same?
>
> How does the similarity/difference of perception affect the group's functioning?

(do's) and proscriptive (don'ts) norms or ground rules that inform interaction at intrapersonal, interpersonal, and systems levels (Nash, 2008). Using normative structures that highlight the commonality of patient-centered care while acknowledging the existence of divergent organizational and personal priorities will help team members to understand that personal goals and wishes will often be subordinate to the goals of the group. The acceptance of professional differences and the proactive examination of errors help to create opportunities for increased communication, understanding, and trust and pave the way for collaborative endeavors between disciplines (Doucet, Larouche, & Melchin, 2001).

As team members come to expect and deliver full participation, and experience consistent adherence to norms associated with role assumption, communication, and authority, accountability is shared. Trust in each other's expertise engenders a parity of participation and shared ownership of team outcomes (Ratcheva, 2009).

Goals

Group goals, like norms, are both explicit and implicit. Implicit goals address the developmental processes inherent to group maturation. Focusing on, defining, and committing to the explicit work-related goals of a group is a major key to success. Commonly held goals and the collective efficacy that the achievements of these goals engender are key contributors to group performance (Silver & Bufanio, 1996). Not surprisingly, the ease of goal attainment is related to the level of goal complexity.

In the current healthcare climate, team goals for professionals are complex and require problem solving using multiple types of data and a convergence of multiple areas of expertise and skill sets. To add to that complexity, interdisciplinary team members bring diverse professional values, individual personal goals, and goals influenced by multiple reporting relationships. It is essential that goals are not only clear but constantly revisited.

Groups that continually communicate and become more explicit with regard to the teams goals are more successful in performance. Regardless of the complexities of the team tasks and team membership, if group members are committed to the group goals, the team can succeed. If the commitment to the goals is low then there is little chance of success (Locke, Latham, & Erez, 1988).

Roles

The inherent diversity of teams makes team members' interaction and relationships key factors in team effectiveness. Researchers have studied groups of people who have a variety of styles in order to ascertain whether a particular complement of individual member styles has any impact on group effectiveness, outcomes, and development. Lewin (1943) observed that behavior is a function of the person and the environment or $B = f$ (P, E). Role assumption in groups is a function of an individual's preferred style or personality in the context of the complex system of group dynamics that comprises team behavior and effectiveness. Subsequent research examined functional roles in groups. These roles are not necessarily attached to any individual but affect the group's developmental progress and productivity.

Wheelan (2005) identifies three primary roles that group members assume regardless of their personality types. Task roles are needed to facilitate a project from inception to completion. Socioemotional or maintenance roles contribute to positive atmosphere of the group and foster cohesion. Organizational roles like the leader, recorder or project manager keep the group organized. According to Benne & Sheats (1948), individual roles

TABLE 3-1   Benne & Sheats's Group Member Roles

Task	Socioemotional/ Maintenance	Individual
Initiator/contributor	Encourager	Aggressor
Information seeker/giver	Harmonizer	Blocker
Coordinator	Compromiser	Disrupter
Evaluator	Includer	Dominator
Energizer	Follower	
Procedural technician		

Data from: Benne, K. & Sheats, P. (1948). Functional roles of group members. *Journal of Social Issues*, 4(2), 41–49.

tend to disrupt group progress and weaken cohesion. **Table 3-1** provides examples of each role.

Belbin (2010) studied teamwork and observed that people in teams tend to assume various team roles, which alternate in their dominance depending upon the developmental stage of the group's activities. The nine roles where categorized into the following three groups: Action oriented, people oriented, and thought oriented. The action-oriented group includes shaper (SH), implementer (IMP), and completer-finisher (CF) roles. The people-oriented group includes coordinator (CO), team worker (TW), and resource investigator (RI) roles. The thought-oriented group includes plant (PL), monitor-evaluator (ME), and specialist (SP) roles. Each team role is associated with typical behavioral and interpersonal strengths. Belbin also defined characteristic weaknesses that tend to accompany each team role. He called these the allowable weaknesses—areas to be aware of and potentially improve upon (see **Table 3-2**).

A group that is composed of members who assume only those roles related to job completion while ignoring the roles that engage and facilitate member participation runs the risk of diminished cohesion, unmanaged conflict, and apathy. All of these negatively affect the sustainability of good performance and successful outcomes. However, groups that are stymied in a quagmire

TABLE 3-2 Belbin's Team Roles

Team Role	Contribution	Allowable Weakness
Thought Oriented (TO)		
Plant	• Creative, imaginative, unorthodox • Solves difficult problems	• Ignores incidentals • Too preoccupied to communicate effectively
Monitor Evaluator	• Sober, strategic, and discerning • Sees all positions • Judges accurately	• Lacks drive and ability to inspire others
Specialist	• Single minded, self-starting, dedicated • Provides knowledge and skills in rare supply	• Contributes on only a narrow front • Dwells on technicalities
Action Oriented (AO)		
Shaper	• Challenging, dynamic • Thrives on pressure • Has the drive and courage to overcome obstacles	• Prone to provocation • Offends people's feelings
Implementer	• Disciplined, reliable, conservative, and efficient • Turns ideas into practical actions	• Somewhat inflexible • Slow to respond to new possibilities
Completer/ Finisher	• Painstaking, conscientious, anxious • Searches out errors and omissions • Polishes and perfects	• Inclined to worry unduly • Reluctant to delegate
People Oriented (PO)		
Team Worker	• Cooperative, mild, perceptive, and diplomatic • Listens • Builds, averts friction	• Indecisive in crunch situations

TABLE 3-2 Belbin's Team Roles *(Continued)*

Team Role	Contribution	Allowable Weakness
Resource Investigator	• Extrovert, enthusiastic, communicative • Explores opportunities • Develops contacts	• Overly optimistic • Loses interest once initial enthusiasm has passed
Coordinator	• Mature, confident; a good chairperson • Clarifies goals, promotes decision making • Delegates well	• Can be seen as manipulative • Offloads personal work

Reproduced with permission from: of Belbin Associates, www.belbin.com.

of conflicting emotions or that are burdened with members who are myopically focused on their personal agenda will never get any work done. These scenarios can negatively impact healthcare teams who routinely deal with issues related to complex medical decision-making and the resultant interventions that will impact a patient's lifestyle and quality of life. Throughout the life of every group of health professionals, leaders and members must be alert enough to recognize what roles need to be assumed and be flexible enough to assume the roles that will sustain optimum group functioning and consistently positive patient outcomes.

The attempt to carry out functional group roles, as described, is further complicated by the many other personal and professional roles that are held by members of healthcare teams. While a primary challenge for all team members is to separate personal needs and roles from the team needs and roles, healthcare professionals must also juggle team and discipline-related roles that often conflict at the intraprofessional and interprofessional levels. Perceived roles and responsibilities may diverge based on variations in professional socialization, experience, and organizational expectations. Some professionals—often from the same discipline—may see themselves as primarily responsible for the physiology of care while others believe they need to incorporate the contextual aspects of the illness experience in their treatment planning (Doucet et al., 2001). When faced with budget restrictions in a rehabilitation department, does the physical therapist on the team focus her energy on advocating for the physical therapy equipment budget or facilitating a group discussion regarding prioritizing the needs of the department? The answer depends on how group, member, and contextual issues are negotiated. Each member of the healthcare team is faced with similar decisions about role choices. These choices will affect the culture, development, and performance of the team and ultimately determine the nature of patient outcomes (Freshman, Rubino, & Chassiakos, 2010).

Communication Patterns

In spite of the role differentiation that exists among the disciplines, holistic approaches to health care can engender role overlap, ambiguity, and boundary management challenges (Gray, 2008; Klein, 2010; Nash, 2008). Teams that leverage common ground as well as disciplinary differences through well-constructed and maintained communication strategies are likely to demonstrate sustained high performance and achieve positive patient outcomes (Drinka & Clark, 2000; Gittel, 2009).

The first step in productive communication is to get the attention of the person with whom one is trying to communicate. Team members who understand that communication styles often reflect learning styles and professional orientation will be most successful if they take the time to adjust their communication style to complement the styles of the people with whom they are communicating. People who are action oriented are interested and tend to talk about objectives, results, performance, and productivity. Strategies, organization, and facts tend to pique the attention of those who are process oriented. People who are idea oriented are interested in concept development and innovation, while those with a people orientation focus their communication on values, beliefs, and relationship building (Youker, 1996).

While the previous examples give an indication of *how* communication is carried out and received, the following model

CASE STUDY: *Communication Style Match*

Members of the interprofessional team on a geriatric unit (physician, nurse, physical therapist, occupational therapist, and social worker) are meeting to discuss patient safety on the unit. During the previous quarter, falls increased by 10%. Analysis of the incident reports indicates that an examination of the fall prevention program that is offered jointly by nursing, physical therapy, and occupational therapy is indicated. The team is meeting with the goal of designing a revised fall prevention program for the unit. The proposed program will need to be based in the most current evidence, ensure the safety of the patients, and be cost effective. All four styles of communication noted previously in this chapter—action oriented (physician and physical therapist), process oriented (occupational therapist), people oriented (social worker), and idea oriented (nurse)—are represented. The leader (in this case, it is the physical therapist) is an identified action-oriented communicator. In preparation for the first meeting, she reviews strategies for adjusting her communication style to the team members and prepares her opening remarks. Her remarks might vary depending on how she perceives the other members of the group. She lists pointers for addressing the others based on their communication styles, along with alternate statements for each type.

COMMUNICATING WITH AN ACTION-ORIENTED PERSON:

- Focus on the results first.
- State your best recommendation.
- Emphasize the practicality of your idea.

At the first meeting, if the other members are action oriented, the physical therapist might say, "The purpose of this group is to address the increased number of falls on the unit this last quarter. We need to revise the fall prevention program that is currently offered. I recommend that we construct a program around the three components that have been identified in the literature. Developing a fall prevention program that includes exercise, fall prevention, and environmental components is the most effective focus."

COMMUNICATING WITH A PROCESS-ORIENTED PERSON:

- State the facts.
- Present your thoughts in a logical manner.

(continues)

- Include options with pros and cons.
- Do not rush the person.

If the other members are process oriented, the physical therapist might say, "The purpose of this group is to address the increased number of falls on the unit this last quarter. We need to revise the fall prevention program that is currently offered. One option that we may choose to pursue is to do a literature review on the efficacy of fall prevention and develop a custom program for our unit. We may also explore the option of purchasing existing modules. What are your thoughts?"

COMMUNICATING WITH A PEOPLE-ORIENTED PERSON:

- Allow for small talk at the beginning of a session.
- Stress the relationship between the proposal and the people concerned.
- Show how the idea worked well in the past.
- Show respect for people.

The physical therapist might say to such a group, "The purpose of this group is to address the increased number of falls on the unit this last quarter. Each of you has been chosen for this team because of your demonstrated commitment to patient safety. You are the experts in the day-to-day care of our patients. One area that we may need to consider is a revision of the fall prevention program that we currently offer. Institutions that are similar to ours have reported great success in reducing patient falls using a combination of exercise, addressing fear of falling, and modifying the environment."

COMMUNICATING WITH AN IDEA-ORIENTED PERSON:

- Allow enough time for discussion.
- Do not get impatient when they go off on tangents.
- Be broad and conceptual in your opening.

The physical therapist could address this type of group by saying, "As key staff members on this geriatric unit, you have demonstrated your commitment to patient safety. I have asked each of you to be a member of this team because we have yet another safety concern. The purpose of this group is to address the increased number of falls on the unit this last quarter. We need to revise the fall prevention program that is currently offered.

Yes, the plan for tornado drills has been effective. Is there anything that we learned during the development and implementation of the tornado drill policy that we can bring to the creation of a fall prevention program?"

By acknowledging the presence of a variety of communication styles and adjusting her approach, this leader has demonstrated respect for team members and hopefully avoided potential problems in team communication at the beginning of this important project.

provides some insight into *what* is communicated. Conscious attention to how and *what* is communicated allows for more mindful, strategic, and effective communication in teams.

The Johari window (Luft & Ingham, 1950) is a classic model for identifying and improving an individual's relationship with a group and/or a group's relationships with other groups. While the discussion that follows addresses the model from an individual perspective, the concepts are applicable to groups as individual entities within organizations, where *others* refers to other groups.

The model is represented as a square that is divided into four window panes or perspectives as shown in **Figure 3-2** and is arranged as follows:

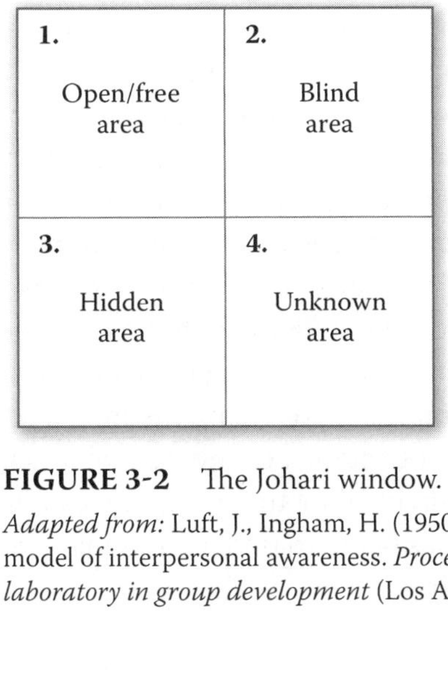

1. Open/free area	2. Blind area
3. Hidden area	4. Unknown area

FIGURE 3-2 The Johari window.

Adapted from: Luft, J., Ingham, H. (1950). The Johari window, a graphic model of interpersonal awareness. *Proceedings of the western training laboratory in group development* (Los Angeles: UCLA).

Quadrant 1: Open/free area—what is known by the individual person and also known by others.

Quadrant 2: Blind area—what is known by others but unknown to the individual.

Quadrant 3: Hidden area—what is known by the individual and consciously hidden from others.

Quadrant 4: Unknown area—what is unknown to both the individual and others.

The panes/areas expand and contract to reflect the proportion of individual or group knowledge about an area. In newly formed groups, for instance, the open area is small since newly assembled groups of people know relatively little about one another. As groups mature, the open area increases as more information is shared and more cooperation and collaboration ensue. If open areas remain diminished, the group may be vulnerable to misunderstanding, mistrust, and confusion and delay progress toward maturity. The ultimate goal for team members is to increase the size of the open area and decrease the size of the other areas through positive communication (see Figure 3-2). The blind area is also known as the "bad breath area" because an individual is unaware of something that is known by everyone else. In the case of an individual, this could be a habit such as constantly glancing at a cell phone during a meeting—unaware that the other members of the group perceive this as disrespectful. Asking for and providing constructive feedback reduce this area.

While it is appropriate to use discretion when disclosing personal or private information, feelings and information related to work proves only be helpful if they are allowed into the open area. The process of disclosure—exposing relevant information and feelings—reduces the hidden area and further expands the open area. So a group member might disclose that he/she feels disrespected when someone is checking a cell phone during a meeting or conversation. The unknown area contains information such as unconscious needs, motivations, or inherent abilities that are unrecognized by the individual or the group. By examining the unknown area, individuals begin to understand that perceptions of present situations may be rooted in our past and the insecurity or anger that may have been experienced during a difficult childhood may be a hot button that is easily triggered by a difficult interaction in the present.

With the realization that our perceptions of present situations are formed through the lens of our own life experiences, we begin to seek information from others in order to construct a more complete picture. The ability to separate our perceptions from actuality allows us to become emotionally independent, no longer bound by automatic negative responses to triggers or hot buttons and better able to make strategic choices regarding our actions and reactions.

If the unknown area is not reduced, the group runs the risk of not being able to leverage all of an individual's talents.

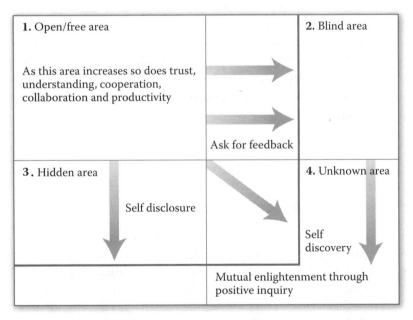

FIGURE 3-3 Detail of the steps involved in a working Johari window.

Data from: Luft, J., Ingham, H. (1950). The Johari window, a graphic model of interpersonal awareness. *Proceedings of the western training laboratory in group development* (Los Angeles: UCLA).

In addition, the individual runs the risk of not realizing his/her true potential—bound by old ways of knowing and reacting and reducing the chances of self-actualization and motivation to become engaged in the group's work. This type of awareness can be sparked through self-discovery, observations by others, and methods of inquiry that encourage mutual discovery. Leaders and members who use positive communication to facilitate self-discovery, solicit and provide constructive feedback, and foster the free flow of information create a psychologically safe environment that engenders creativity, productivity, and sustained high performance.

Leavitt (1951) described graphic configurations of the most common communication networks in small groups such as the wheel and circle. An important aspect of communication networks is how information is processed and distributed. Simple tasks that require the processing of limited amounts of information are most efficiently carried out in centralized networks like the wheel where one person serves as the hub for information exchange, while more complex tasks, which require the processing of large amounts of complex information, are most efficiently handled by decentralized networks of communication such as the circle, where there is a free flowing information exchange among all participants.

COMMUNICATION NETWORKS

Simple tasks, like stocking supply closets in the therapy gyms, requires the processing of limited amounts of information and can be most efficiently carried out in a centralized network like the wheel. A supervisor (hub of the wheel) might send out a directive to the therapy aides. More complex tasks, like developing a comprehensive patient discharge plan, requires the processing of large amounts of complex information and might be most efficiently handled by decentralized networks of communication between the physician, nurse, therapists, and social worker.

(continues)

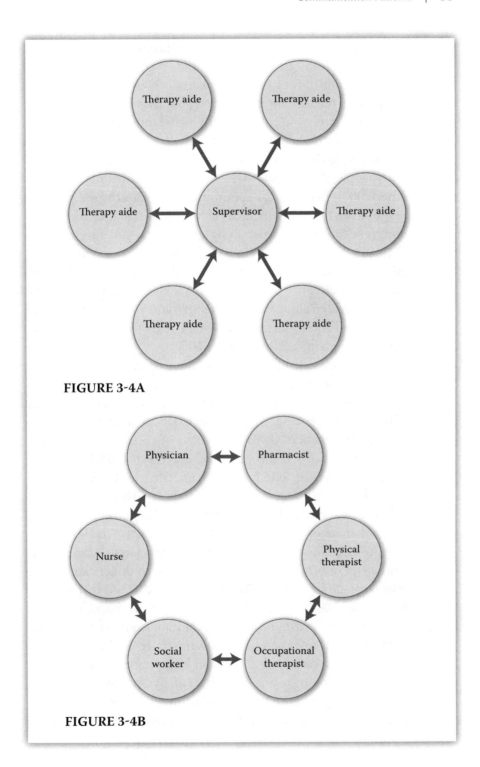

FIGURE 3-4A

FIGURE 3-4B

Systematic observation of communication and attraction patterns provides insight into morale and levels of satisfaction flow of information, power and influence, cohesiveness, and effectiveness within teams. Communication patterns tend to parallel role, status, and attraction patterns with higher interaction rates being associated with higher status individuals. Lower status individuals are less likely to express their thoughts and feelings in groups with people of higher status. According to the Institutes of Medicine (2003), hierarchical communication patterns are partially responsible for many medical errors. Additional challenges to communication may exist along gender and generational lines (Spector, 2010). However, in teams that continually employ collaborative processes characterized by directness, mutual understanding, and parity of participation, a climate of psychological safety is created along with an effective and efficient exchange of information among all members of the team (Meads & Ashcroft, 2005; Nembhard & Edmondson, 2006.

Healthcare organizations are composed of a diverse network of health professionals, patients, and caregivers who must leverage each other's expertise by coordinating the exchange and flow of highly complex data. High-quality feedback among interdependent team members yields high levels of cohesion, satisfaction, and performance in teams (Garman, 2010; Gittell, 2009; Goleman, Boyatzis & McKee, 2002). To this end, conscious effort must be applied to developing information exchange strategies that distribute leadership and facilitate accountability and engagement of every member of the team (Gray, 2008; Hammick, Freeth, Copperman, & Goodsman, 2009). Attention to the analysis of social networks and information exchange is crucial to understanding the interpersonal aspects of collaboration around a task, goal, or function (Gray, 2008). Social and interpersonal processes, including team members' collaborative styles, communication networks, and conflict management and negotiation strategies that emphasize excellence and convey clear goals and expectations are hallmarks of high-functioning teams (Stokols, Hall, Tylor, & Moser, 2008).

The fast-paced healthcare environment places time at a premium. Managers and practitioners find it difficult to justify taking time away from direct patient care in order to attend meetings. However, recent healthcare reforms have linked reimbursement to patient outcomes such as length of stay, readmission rates, and patient satisfaction rather than the number of procedures and services provided. High-functioning healthcare teams have been associated with positive patient outcomes and high retention rates for health professionals. While one could argue that the time spent in meetings is not reimbursable, it would be hard to deny that the improvements in team communication and performance positively affect team sustainability and patient outcomes. Institutions that invest in the development of relationships through formal structures that support frequent and consistent time allocation for team interaction—face-to-face and electronic—will find that gains in patient outcomes will mirror gains in social capital (Drinka & Clark, 2000; Ghaye, 2005; Gittell, 2009; IOM, 2003; Lawrence, 2002; Ratcheva, 2009).

CASE STORY: *Check Your Ego at the Door*

Any complicated problem lends itself to an interprofessional approach. When we have to do any project we have groups where there are 12 people in different areas on the team (eg: graphics, engineering, administration, nursing) and they talk about the project. Then we break the team into smaller groups of 3 and they all have to come back with their proposed designs and talk about the process of coming to that conclusion. The group, as a whole, reviews all the alternative proposals and pulls them together for their final decision. No one person has the final say—it is not hierarchical. This fosters the idea that everyone has something to contribute. Everyone understands that you have to check your ego at the door. It is not about you. The final decision reflects the goals of the program, not individual goals.

This approach is neither intuitive or the individualistic "American way." There should be some kind of training so that people learn how to separate their work performance from their own personal needs and work as a team.

—Karen J. Nichols, Chief Medical Officer, University of Pennsylvania LIFE (Living Independently for Elders) Program

REFLECTION: *Recognizing and Respecting Diversity*

How do you demonstrate respect of diversity in the healthcare team?

How might you use conflict as a path to creative problem solving in the healthcare team?

How do you find shared ground?

How do you influence others on your team?

How do they influence you?

Collaborative, participative environments engender increased knowledge and respect of the health team members for each other. Increased awareness of the expertise available to the team will facilitate the team's ability to distribute leadership based on the nature of the challenge, or problem and disciplinary boundaries can become points of connection and innovation rather than points of contention (Drinka & Clark, 2000; Gray, 2008; Meads & Ashcroft, 2005; Wheatley, 2006). Leaders, who are willing to trust in the diverse wisdom and singular intent of the collective, actively encourage, and seek participation from all members of the team. Consequently, communication disparities are mitigated and psychologically safe team environments are created. All members are encouraged to contribute, exercise leadership, and be personally engaged and accountable for the team outcomes. (Nembhard & Edmondson, 2006; Wheatley, 2006).

References

Belbin, R. (2010). *Team Roles at work* (2nd ed.). Burlington, MA: Butterworth Heinemann/Elsevier.

Benne, K., & Sheats, P. (1948). Functional roles of group members. *Journal of Social Issues, 4*(2), 41–49.

Doucet, H., Larouche, J., & Melchin, K. (2001). *Ethical deliberation in multiprofessional health care teams*. Ottawa, Canada: University of Ottawa Press.

Drinka, T., & Clark, P. (2000). *Health care teamwork: Interdisciplinary practice and teaching*. Westport, CT: Auburn House.

Freshman, B., Rubino, L., & Chassiakos, Y. (2010). *Collaboration across the disciplines in health care*. Sudbury, MA: Jones and Bartlett Learning.

Garman, A. (2010). Leadership development in the interdisciplinary context. In F. Freshman, L. Rubino, & Y. Chassiakos (Eds.), *Collaboration across the disciplines in health care* (pp. 43–64). Sudbury, MA: Jones and Bartlett Learning.

Ghaye, T. (2005). *Developing the reflective healthcare team*. Oxford, UK: Blackwell Publishing, Ltd.

Gittell, J. (2009). *High performance healthcare: Using the power of relationships to achieve quality, efficiency and resilience*. New York, NY: McGraw-Hill.

Goleman, D., Boyatzis, R., & McKee, A. (2002). *Primal leadership: Learning to lead with emotional intelligence*. Boston, MA: Harvard Business School Press.

Gray, B. (2008). Enhancing transdisciplinary research through collaborative leadership. *American Journal of Preventative Medicine, 35*(2S), 124–132.

Hammick, M., Freeth, D., Copperman, J., & Goodsman, D. (2009). *Being interprofessional*. Malden, MA: Polity Press.

Institutes of Medicine, Committee on Quality of Health Care in America, National Academy of Sciences. (2003). *Health professions education: A bridge to quality*. Washington, DC: National Academy Press.

Klein, J. (2010). *Creating interdisciplinary campus cultures: A model for strength and sustainability*. San Francisco, CA: Jossey-Bass.

Lawrence, D. (2002). *From chaos to care: The promise of team based medicine*. Cambridge, MA: Perseus Publishing.

Leavitt, H. (1951). Some effects of certain communication patterns on group performance. *Journal of Abnormal and Social Psychology, 46*, 38–50.

Lewin, K. (1943). Defining the "field at a given time." *Psychological Review, 50*, 292–310.

Locke, E. A., Latham, G. P., & Erez, M. (1988). The determinants of goal commitment. *Academy of Management Review, 1*, 23–39.

Luft, J., & Ingham, H. (1950). The Johari window, a graphic model of interpersonal awareness. *Proceedings of the Western Training Laboratory in Group Development.* Los Angeles, CA: UCLA.

Meads, G., & Ashcroft, J. (2005). *The case for interprofessional collaboration in health and social care.* Oxford, UK: Blackwell Publishing, Ltd.

Nash, J. (2008). Transdisciplinary training: Key components and prerequisites for success. *American Journal of Preventative Medicine, 35*(2S), s133–s140.

Nembhard, I., & Edmondson, A. (2006). Making it safe: The effects of leader inclusiveness and professional status on psychological safety and improvement efforts in health care teams. *Journal of Organizational Behavior, 27*, 941–966.

O'Daniel, M., & Rosenstein, A. H. (2008, April). Professional communication and team collaboration. In R. G. Hughes (Ed.), *Patient safety and quality: An evidence-based handbook for nurses* (Chapter 33). Rockville, MD: Agency for Healthcare Research and Quality. Retrieved from http://www.ncbi.nlm. nih.gov/books/NBK2637/

Ratcheva, V. (2009). Integrating diverse knowledge through boundary spanning processes: The case for multidisciplinary project teams. *International Journal of Project Management, 27*, 206–215.

Sherif, M. (1936). *The psychology of social norms.* New York, NY: Harper & Row.

Silver, W., & Bufanio, K. (1996, August). The impact of group efficacy and group goals on group task performance. *Small Group Research, 27*, 347–359.

Spector, N. (2010). Interprofessional collaboration: A nursing perspective. In F. Freshman, L. Rubino, & Y. Chassiakos (Eds.), *Collaboration across the disciplines in healthcare* (pp. 107). Sudbury, MA: Jones and Bartlett Learning.

Stokols, D., Hall, K., Tylor, B., & Moser, R. (2008). The science of team science. *American Journal of Preventative Medicine, 35*(2S), s77–s89.

Torrens, P. (2010). The health care team members: Who are they and what do they do? In F. Freshman, L. Rubino, & Y.

Chassiakos (Eds.), *Collaboration across the disciplines in health care* (pp. 1–19). Sudbury, MA: Jones and Bartlett.

Wheatley, M. (2006). *Leadership and the new science: Discovering order in a chaotic world* (3rd ed.). San Francisco, CA: Berrett-Koehler Publishers, Inc.

Wheelan, S. (2005). *Group process: A developmental perspective* (2nd ed.). Needham Heights, MA: Allyn & Bacon.

Youker, R. (1996). Communication style instrument: A team building tool. In *PMI Seminars & Symposium Proceedings* (pp. 796–799). Upper Darby, PA: Project Management Institute.

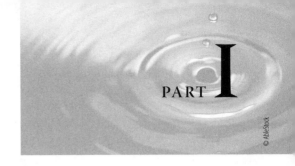

PART I

Team and Group Development Activities

Activity 1: How Much of a Team Is Your Group?

In chapter 1, the difference between a group and a team is described on a continuum. At one end, a "group" refers to any group of people with something in common and at the other end of the spectrum, "team" refers to people who must work together to reach a common goal or outcome. Identify three groups or teams that you have been a part of. Place them on a continuum and provide a rationale for your decision.

Activity 2: *I* and *We*

From your experience as a member or leader in an interprofessional team, develop two cases to analyze from the "I" and the "We" perspective. Specifically, identify those times when you:

- Made a decision in the team's interest and not your interest. What was the effect on you? On the members of the team?
- Made a decision in the patient's interest and not your interest. What was the effect on you? On the patient?

Activity 3: TOPS: Team Orientation and Performance Survey

TOPS is a survey that can help you determine where the energy of the group is focused. When you fill this out, remember that this is your perception of the team. Other team members may see it differently. Rank the endings of each sentence according to how well each ending describes your team. Enter a 4 for the sentence ending that *best* describes your team now, down to a 1 for the sentence ending that seems *least* like your team. Be sure to rank all the endings for each sentence unit.

Utilizing the scores on the TOPS, refer to the text for a description of the developmental level that is most like your team. At which group developmental stage is your team? Is the TOPS score consistent with your experience of the team? What strategies could you use as a team member or leader to positively impact the team's development?

1. Team members:	___ talk about topics that are safe.	___ argue with each other.	___ are open with the group about their thoughts and feelings.	___ talk openly about issues and concerns and give constructive feedback.
2. Team members:	___ tend to agree.	___ disagree with each other.	___ offer relevant facts, opinions, and ideas during group discussions.	___ resolve conflicts before moving on to other subjects.
3. Team members:	___ don't voice differences of opinion.	___ don't handle conflicts constructively.	___ can be candid about differences of opinion.	___ listen to different points of view and use the differences to create more effective outcomes.
4. Team members:	___ depend on the leader for direction.	___ depend on the leader for direction yet resent the direction the leader gives.	___ utilize the leader as an advisor, and the leader delegates responsibility for process, decisions, and implementation to the team.	___ share the leadership function.
5. Team members:	___ direct almost all comments toward the leader.	___ vary in their support of the leader.	___ have a positive evaluation of the leader's abilities.	___ recognize and utilize the leader for his or her strengths.

6. Team members:	___ do not disagree with the leader.	___ tend to disagree with the leader.	___ trust that the leader is giving them the information and authority they need to get the job done.	___ see the leader as a resource to help them get the job done.
7. Team members:	___ have a purpose and goals that are unclear.	___ disagree about goals.	___ agree about the team goals.	___ have goals that are well defined and measurable.
8. Team members:	___ have roles that are unclear.	___ are confused about roles, tasks, and responsibilities.	___ have role assignments that are defined and match their abilities.	___ understand each other's roles, and they are not overly rigid.
9. The team:	___ has a structure and processes that are organized by the leader.	___ feels disorganized.	___ is talking about and agreeing on how to organize work.	___ is well organized and can adjust processes and procedures to fit the work task.
10. Team members:	___ are concerned with being liked.	___ want recognition for the unique skills and abilities they bring to the team.	___ behave with trust, respect, and caring toward one another and what they bring to the team.	___ have a *we* orientation rather than a *me* orientation.
11. Team members:	___ do not feel like a team.	___ have expressed frustration within the group.	___ communicate appreciation for each other's talents and capabilities.	___ are safe for taking interpersonal risk.

12. Team members:	___ are concerned with fitting in.	___ feel tension in the group.	___ trust each other's intentions.	___ can implement decisions that are best for the team as a whole even if they conflict with individual preferences.
Totals	DI =	CC =	TS =	WP =

DI = dependency and inclusion; CC = counterdependency and conflict; TS = trust and structure; WP = energy in work and productivity.

Source: Developed by Felice Tilin for GroupWorks Consulting, LLC (owned by Felice Tilin) 2009 Felice Tilin. All rights reserved.

Activity 4: Team Goal Setting

The most effective team goals are specific, measurable, attainable, relevant, and time bound (SMART). The following questions will help you and your team to create SMART goals. Think of a short-term project that is important for your team to accomplish. Use these questions to inform your goal development and evaluate whether your goals have been achieved.

- What goals does the organization expect this team to achieve?
- Can we operationally define the goal(s)?
- Are the goals clear to each member of the team?
- Does it tell the team who, what, when, where, which, and why?
  - *What:* What do we want to accomplish?
  - *Why:* Specific reasons, purpose, or benefits of accomplishing the goal.
  - *Who:* Who is involved?
  - *Where and when:* Identify locations and time lines.
  - *Which:* Identify requirements and constraints.

Measurable

What are the criteria for measuring progress toward the attainment of the goal? Measuring keeps a team on track, helps the team reach its target dates, and tests whether it has completed tasks, milestones, and final accomplishments.

A measurable goal will usually answer questions such as:

- How much?
- How many?
- When?

Attainable

Are the goals realistic and attainable? Does the team have the right members on it to do the job (or can it recruit these members?). Does the team have resources and the proper amount of authority? Who are the champions in the organization? How will the team get help when it needs it?

An attainable goal will usually answer the question:

- *How:* How can the goal be accomplished?

Relevant

- Who is this important to? Goals that are relevant to the superiors, the team, or the organization should receive that needed support.
- How is it relevant to each individual on the team?
- How does it support or align with other organizational goals?
- How does it align with an overall organizational strategy, organizational values, and/or its mission?

A relevant goal can answer yes to these questions:

- Is it worthwhile?
- Is this the right time?
- Does this match our other efforts/needs?
- Are we the right people to get this job one?

Time Bound

What is the target for completion? When will the team complete tasks, mini goals, and milestones? This part of the SMART goal criteria is intended to prevent goals from being overtaken by the day-to-day crises that invariably arise in an organization. A time-bound goal is intended to establish a sense of urgency.

A time-bound goal will usually answer the questions:

- When?
- What can we do in 10 days, 10 weeks, and 10 months?
- What do we need to accomplish today?

Source: Developed by Felice Tilin for GroupWorks Consulting, LLC (owned by Felice Tilin) 2000 Felice Tilin. All rights reserved.

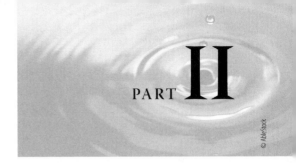

Relationship-Centered Leadership

"If your actions inspire others to dream more, do more and become more . . . you are a leader."

John Quincy Adams

Chapter 4: Perspectives on Leadership

Chapter 5: Leadership Building Blocks

Chapter 6: Relational Leadership

Part II Activities

CHAPTER **4**

Perspectives on Leadership

Learning Objectives

1. Analyze various theories of leadership.
2. Understand the relationship of personality and leadership styles.
3. Analyze how leadership is affected by the context and situation in which it is exercised.
4. Understand the relationship of emotional intelligence and leadership.
5. Analyze competencies required for health professions leadership.
6. Identify personal leadership characteristics.

Leadership emerges as a compilation of mysteries that have been investigated for centuries. Researchers have attempted to answer questions such as: Are leaders born? Can leaders be developed? Does the environment create the leader? Is leadership emergence synonymous with leader effectiveness? What role does social dynamics have in the leadership equation? Can leadership be shared (Avolio, 2007; Zaccaro, 2007)? How and why should members assume a leadership stance? The latter questions resonate when contemplating the development and sustainability of effective interdisciplinary healthcare teams. An examination of the broader phenomenon of leadership provides a context for that inquiry.

71

Perspectives on Leadership

Leadership connotes position as well as action. Positional leadership refers to responsibility given to an individual or group of individuals to guide, direct, or control. The act of leadership or ability to lead refers to the effective use of influence and a complex dynamic that has inspired much of the research on leadership. Leadership can be simply defined as the exercise of power and influence with others. Some theorists have posited that leaders are born while others focus on the role that social, cultural, political, and environmental factors have on the emergence of leaders.

Many perspectives regarding leadership offer intriguing views of the leadership concept, but no definitive conceptualization exists. A comprehensive review of these views is beyond the scope of this book. For the purposes of our discussion, we will focus on three broad theoretical approaches that are supported by modern-day research and are most applicable to healthcare leadership development. These include personality/trait, contingency/situational, and relational theories. We will provide a summary of each of these theoretical approaches, highlight the most relevant theoretical concepts, and provide opportunities for the practical application of these concepts.

Personality and Trait Theories

Early conceptualizations of leadership focused on the "great man" theory, which hypothesized that leaders were born with certain characteristics that predisposed them to take command and lead others (Carlyle, 1841). The Zeitgeist theory credited the convergence of social, political and individual factors with the emergence of a leader—the right person for the right time in history (Tolstoy, 1869). Subsequent trait theorists, informed by the big five theory of personality (discussed later in this chapter), described a constellation of traits that were indicative of a leadership personality.

MYERS-BRIGGS TYPE INDICATOR

One of the first and most widely used models to identify traits was developed by Katharine Cook Briggs and Isabel Briggs Myers based on the Carl Jung's psychological type theory. Jung's theory is based on a hypothesis that people are born with innate personality traits (Jung, 1991; Myers, McCaulley, Quenk & Hammer, 1998).

The Myers-Briggs type indicator (MBTI) is a self-report survey instrument that helps to determine personality and preferred behavioral style across the following four dichotomies: extroversion/introversion, sensing/intuition, thinking/feeling, and judging/perceiving. The MBTI is designed to determine preferences for finding energy, gathering information, making decisions, and orienting to the environment. While it does not identify talents, quantify intelligence, or predict leadership success, it facilitates self-awareness, which does correlate with leadership success (Goleman & Boyatzis, 2008).

MYERS-BRIGGS TYPE DICHOTOMIES

This diagram summarizes the four types of dichotomies and their related preferences based on Myers and Briggs's conceptualization.

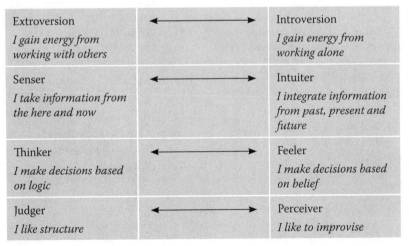

Extroversion		Introversion
I gain energy from working with others	←——————→	*I gain energy from working alone*
Senser		Intuiter
I take information from the here and now	←——————→	*I integrate information from past, present and future*
Thinker		Feeler
I make decisions based on logic	←——————→	*I make decisions based on belief*
Judger		Perceiver
I like structure	←——————→	*I like to improvise*

Data from: Myers, Isabel Briggs; McCaulley Mary H., Quenk, Naomi L., Hammer, Allen L. (1998). MBTI Manual (*A guide to the development and use of the Myers Briggs type indicator*). Consulting Psychologists Press; 3rd ed.

REFLECTION: *MBTI Detailed Descriptions*

Read the following descriptions to determine your personality and preferred behavioral style on each of the four MBTI dichotomies.

Extroversion/Introversion—How a Person Finds Energy	
Extroverts (E) are energized by the outside world (people and things).	Introverts (I) are energized by being alone with their internal thoughts.
• Draw energy from action • Tend to act first, then reflect, and then act again • Energy level tends to drop when not engaged in an activity • Are influenced by the expectations and attention of others • Enjoy working in groups	• Draw energy from reflection • Prefer to reflect before acting • Energy tends to drop with too much external interaction • May defend against external demands and intrusions • Enjoy working alone or with a few others

Sensing/Intuiting—How a Person Takes in Information	
Sensors (S) prefer to take in information in the here and now and in a precise manner.	Intuitives (N) like to take in information in a holistic and extemporaneous manner.
• Focus on objective facts and circumstances as perceived by the senses (seeing, feeling, hearing) first • Have excellent powers of observation • Deal with how things are rather than on how they could be • See problems as needing specific solutions based on past information • Value realism	• Focus on the big picture and underlying pattern, beyond the reach of the senses first • Have vivid powers of imagination • Focus more on how things could be rather than how they are • See problems as opportunities to innovate based on inspiration • Value imagination

Thinking/Feeling—How a Person Prefers to Make a Decision	
Thinkers (T) will choose objectivity and logic when making decisions	Feelers (F) will choose what they believe in when they make a decision.
• Seek logic and clarity	• Seek emotional clarity
• Question first	• Accept first
• Have an interest in data	• Have an interest in people
• Know when logic is required	• Know when support is required
• Prefer objectivity	• Consider impact on people
• Weigh pros and cons	• Weigh values
• Strive to be fair	• Strive to be compassionate

Judging/Perceiving—How a Person Prefers to Live His/Her Life	
Judging (J) types like to come to closure and take action.	Perceiving (P) types like to remain open and adapt to new information.
• Prefer matters to be settled and structured	• Prefer things to be flexible and open
• Finish before deadline	• Finish task at the deadline
• Like plans and goals and reducing surprises	• Like to see what turns up and enjoy surprises
• Quickly commit to a plan	• Reserve the right to change a plan
• See routines as effective	• See routines as limiting
• Trust the plan	• Trust the process

REFLECTION: *MBTI 16 Types at a Glance*

Read the following descriptions and match your MBTI findings to interpret your personality and preferred behavioral style on each of the four MBTI dichotomies.

The 16 MBTI Types

ISTJ (Introversion, Sensing, Thinking, Judging)

Quiet, serious, earn success by thoroughness and dependability. Practical, matter-of-fact, realistic, and responsible. Decide logically what should be done and work toward it steadily, regardless of distractions. Take pleasure in making everything orderly and organized—their work, their home, their life. Value traditions and loyalty.

ISFJ (Introversion, Sensing, Feeling, Judging)

Quiet, friendly, responsible, and conscientious. Committed and steady in meeting their obligations. Thorough, painstaking, and accurate. Loyal, considerate, notice and remember specifics about people who are important to them, concerned with how others feel. Strive to create an orderly and harmonious environment at work and at home.

INFJ (Introversion, Intuitive, Feeling, Judging)

Seek meaning and connection in ideas, relationships, and material possessions. Want to understand what motivates people and are insightful about others. Conscientious and committed to their firm values. Develop a clear vision about how best to serve the common good. Organized and decisive in implementing their vision.

INTJ (Introversion, Intuitive, Thinking, Judging)

Have original minds and great drive for implementing their ideas and achieving their goals. Quickly see patterns in external events and develop long-range explanatory perspectives. When committed, organize a job and carry it through. Skeptical and independent, have high standards of competence and performance—for themselves and others.

ISTP (Introversion, Sensing, Thinking, Perceiving)

Tolerant and flexible, quiet observers until a problem appears, then act quickly to find workable solutions. Analyze what makes things work and readily get through large amounts of data to isolate the core of practical problems. Interested in cause and effect, organize facts using logical principles, value efficiency.

(continues)

ISFP (Introversion, Sensing, Feeling, Perceiving)

Quiet, friendly, sensitive, and kind. Enjoy the present moment, what's going on around them. Like to have their own space and to work within their own time frame. Loyal and committed to their values and to people who are important to them. Dislike disagreements and conflicts, do not force their opinions or values on others.

INFP (Introversion, Intuitive, Feeling, Perceiving)

Idealistic, loyal to their values and to people who are important to them. Want an external life that is congruent with their values. Curious, quick to see possibilities, can be catalysts for implementing ideas. Seek to understand people and to help them fulfill their potential. Adaptable, flexible, and accepting unless a value is threatened.

INTP (Introversion, Intuitive, Thinking, Perceiving)

Seek to develop logical explanations for everything that interests them. Theoretical and abstract, interested more in ideas than in social interaction. Quiet, contained, flexible, and adaptable. Have unusual ability to focus in depth to solve problems in their area of interest. Skeptical, sometimes critical, always analytical.

ESTP (Extroversion, Sensing, Thinking, Perceiving)

Flexible and tolerant, they take a pragmatic approach focused on immediate results. Theories and conceptual explanations bore them—they want to act energetically to solve the problem. Focus on the here-and-now, spontaneous, enjoy each moment that they can be active with others. Enjoy material comforts and style. Learn best through doing.

ESFP (Extroversion, Sensing, Feeling, Perceiving)

Outgoing, friendly, and accepting. Exuberant lovers of life, people, and material comforts. Enjoy working with others to make things happen. Bring common sense and a realistic approach to their work, and make work fun. Flexible and spontaneous, adapt readily to new people and environments. Learn best by trying a new skill with other people.

ENFP (Extroversion, Intuitive, Feeling, Perceiving)

Warmly enthusiastic and imaginative. See life as full of possibilities. Make connections between events and information very quickly, and confidently proceed based on the patterns they see. Want a lot of affirmation from others, and readily give appreciation and support. Spontaneous and flexible, often rely on their ability to improvise and their verbal fluency.

(continues)

ENTP (Extroversion, Intuitive, Thinking, Perceiving)

Quick, ingenious, stimulating, alert, and outspoken. Resourceful in solving new and challenging problems. Adept at generating conceptual possibilities and then analyzing them strategically. Good at reading other people. Bored by routine, will seldom do the same thing the same way, apt to turn to one new interest after another.

ESTJ (Extroversion, Sensing, Thinking, Judging)

Practical, realistic, matter-of-fact. Decisive, quickly move to implement decisions. Organize projects and people to get things done, focus on getting results in the most efficient way possible. Take care of routine details. Have a clear set of logical standards, systematically follow them and want others to also. Forceful in implementing their plans.

ESFJ (Extroversion, Sensing, Feeling, Judging)

Warmhearted, conscientious, and cooperative. Want harmony in their environment, work with determination to establish it. Like to work with others to complete tasks accurately and on time. Loyal, follow through even in small matters. Notice what others need in their day-by-day lives and try to provide it. Want to be appreciated for who they are and for what they contribute.

ENFJ (Extroversion, Intuitive, Feeling, Judging)

Warm, empathetic, responsive, and responsible. Highly attuned to the emotions, needs, and motivations of others. Find potential in everyone, want to help others fulfill their potential. May act as catalysts for individual and group growth. Loyal, responsive to praise and criticism. Sociable, facilitate others in a group, and provide inspiring leadership.

ENTJ (Extroversion, Intuitive, Thinking, Judging)

Frank, decisive, assume leadership readily. Quickly see illogical and inefficient procedures and policies, develop and implement comprehensive systems to solve organizational problems. Enjoy long-term planning and goal setting. Usually well informed, well read, enjoy expanding their knowledge and passing it on to others. Forceful in presenting their ideas.

BIG FIVE THEORY OF PERSONALITY

The big five theory of personality suggests that there are five universal personality traits: extroversion (positive attitude, sociable), agreeableness (accommodating, adaptable), conscientiousness (goal oriented), neuroticism (need for stability, pessimistic), and openness (imaginative, creative, open minded). Each of these traits is represented as a continuum that ranges between two extremes (e.g., extroversion and introversion) (McCrae & Costa, 1987). It is accepted that personality is a complex phenomenon with wide variation among individuals. However, according to this theory, the "ideal leader" is resilient (low on the neuroticism factor), energetic and outgoing (high on the extroversion factor), visionary (high on the openness factor), competitive (low on the agreeableness factor), and dedicated to a goal (high on the conscientiousness factor).

Contingency and Situational Theories and Leadership Styles

Contingency and situational theories postulate that effective leaders use a combination of behaviors or styles that are contingent upon the particular situation, the personalities involved, the task, and the organizational culture (Fiedler, 1967; Hersey, 1985). Contingency and situational theorists such as Fiedler (1978) and Hersey and Blanchard (1976, 1982) refrained from describing an ideal leadership style based solely on traits or personality and emphasized that successful leaders are able to understand their motivations and preferred style and are able to adapt their style to the situation and the needs of the group. Fiedler's (1978) basic premise was that leadership was a function of the leader's motivational style and the control requirements of the situation. According to the contingency theory, there are two primary motivations for leaders: relationship building and task completion. In addition, the control requirements of situations are dependent upon leader–member relations, task structure, and positional power. Leader–member relations pertain to the way followers feel about the leader. Tasks can be clearly structured or ambiguous and unstructured. Disinfecting equipment in the physical therapy clinic after a patient treatment session is an example of a highly structured task, while creating a process that will improve patient care in a particular unit from intake to exit would be considered an unstructured task.

Position power is related to the assigned power the leader has over the group. A leader has more positional power if everyone formally reports to that leader. The attending physician has strong positional power over a group of medical residents while a case manager has less positional power over the nurses and therapists who are part of a treatment team since each of the members report to different units in the organization.

Stress and anxiety increases when the leader's style does not match a situation, and poor decision making is often the result. The most successful outcomes occur when the leader's preferred style matches the situational requirements and they are able to expand their behavioral repertoire through formal training. Relationship-oriented leaders are able to incorporate task-oriented behaviors while task-oriented leaders demonstrate increased relationship-building behaviors (Fiedler, 1978; Northouse, 2010).

Hersey and Blanchard's situational theory (1976, 1982) posits that the best leaders are able shift their focus over time from task to relationships based on the developmental needs of the group. Newly formed or immature groups that have yet to build commitment and expertise may do best with a directive, task-oriented leader, while moderately mature and mature groups are most successful when guided by a supportive, relationship-oriented leader. Ultimately, the level of engagement, participation, autonomy, and maturity that is achieved by the group depends, in part, on the degree to which decision-making authority is shared between the leader and the group members (Blanchard, Zigarmi & Zigarmi, 1985).

Blake and Mouton (1978, 1980, 1982) proposed that leadership style is informed by the degree to which the individual is concerned with task completion or relationship building. Their leadership grid provided a graphic representation of the variations in leadership styles ranging from (1,1) apathetic and not concerned with people or outcomes to (9,9) a leader who demonstrates his/her dual concern for relationship and goal attainment by fostering teamwork. Blake and Mouton identified the latter as the ideal leadership style.

REFLECTION

The following grid is based on the work of Blake and Mouton (1978, 1980, 1982) and depicts managerial style based on the level of caring about people (concern for people) and caring about getting the job done (concern for production).

1. In the culture of your organization, which style is the most common?

2. Is this style effective? Why or why not?

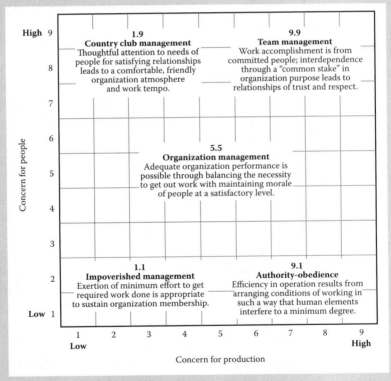

FIGURE 4-1 The leadership grid.

Reproduced from: Blake, R. Moulton, J. (1964). *The Managerial Grid: The Key to Leadership Excellence.* Houston, TX: Gulf Publishing Company.

Relational Theories

Later theories recognized leadership as a reciprocal interaction between leaders and followers with the hallmark of good leadership being transformation of the followers who are committed to the leader's vision (Bass & Avolio, 1994). The application of neuropsychological and neurocognitive research to the field of leadership has supplemented the wealth of information from the sociopsychological fields. Most recently, leadership is conceptualized as a set of learnable attitudes, behaviors, and skills geared toward relationship building. The effect on others is an awakening of self-efficacy, confidence, and capability, which enables proactive, engaged collective action toward a common goal (Goleman et al, 2002).

Emotional Intelligence

Decades of neuropsychological research have established that emotions can dictate our thinking, motivate us, and mobilize us into action. It is generally accepted that thoughts can induce emotions, and emotions also generate thoughts. For instance, when an individual is upset about something (emotion), he or she may engage in self-talk or internal dialogue (thoughts), which may fuel a spiral of intense emotions and upsetting thoughts.

The thoughts and emotions that shape human behavior originate from separate centers of the brain and are interactive determinants of one another. The amygdala or the feeling mind is a primitive part of the brain that triggers a fight-or-flight response, which is tempered by the prefrontal cortex or thinking mind. When stress, drugs, or alcohol compromises the nervous system, the tempering function of the prefrontal cortex may fail to block the instructions from the amygdala, and behavior that is not rational or adaptive to the situation may result.

Effective leaders are not as susceptible to this "amygdala highjack" as other leaders are. They are tuned in to their emotional skills and are able to use them in an appropriate way and in the proper context (Goleman et al, 2002). Daniel Goleman found that outstanding leaders were judged by their superiors as performing significantly better on a constellation of personal skills and social skills that fell into the following four broad categories: self-awareness, self-management, social awareness, and relationship management. This constellation of behaviors has been termed *emotional intelligence* (see **Table 4-1**) and is a prerequisite for relationship building that is the bedrock of sustainable leadership practices (Goleman, 1995). Developing competency in relationship management is contingent upon competency in self-awareness, self-management, and social awareness and essential for success in life and/or workplace.

In most healthcare organizations, leaders and managers are often appointed based on expertise and years of experience. However, as supervisory responsibility increases, so does the need for people-handling skills. Research indicates that some leaders and managers who are appointed primarily because of technical skill

TABLE 4-1 Emotional Intelligence Domains

Self-Awareness: The ability of an individual to be cognizant of his/her own emotions, acknowledge personal strengths and weaknesses and describe how emotions impact his/her actions. Self-awareness includes the emotional self-awareness competency and is highly correlated with accurate self-assessment and self-confidence.

Self-Management: The ability to moderate negative emotional responses, to remain calm in stressful situations, adapt to change, continually work to improve oneself and stay optimistic in challenging situations. Competencies include achievement orientation, adaptability, emotional self-control and positive outlook.

Social Awareness: The ability to understand other individuals, teams and organizations by being open to other perspectives, putting oneself in another person's shoes, understanding the values, culture and unspoken rules in a team or organization. The competencies included are empathy and organizational awareness.

Relationship Management: The ability to constructively resolve conflicts, coach and mentor others, inspire others by expressing a compelling vision, strategically influence others and to work as an effective member of a team. These competencies include skills in conflict management, coaching and mentoring, influencing, inspirational leadership and teambuilding.

Adapted from: Goleman, D., Boyatzis, R. and McKee, A. (2002). *Primal Leadership: Realizing the Power of Emotional Intelligence*. Boston, MA: Harvard Business School Press.

REFLECTION: *Emotional Intelligence Checklist*

Rate yourself on each of the components of the emotional intelligence checklist to determine your characteristics in each of the domains.

Emotional Intelligence Checklist	
SELF-AWARENESS	
Emotional self-awareness: Recognizing how our emotions affect our performance	One who has emotional self-awareness: • Is aware of one's own feelings and can speak openly about them • Can identify the triggers to and inner signals of his or her own emotions • Recognizes the effects of one's own feelings on one's behavior • Displays emotional insight, seeing the big picture in a complex situation
Accurate self-assessment: Knowing one's own inner resources, abilities and limits	One who makes an accurate self-assessment: • Is aware of his or her own strengths and limitations • Welcomes honest, constructive criticism and is open to feedback • Has a sense of humor about oneself • Knows when to seek assistance
Self-confidence: A strong sense of one's self-worth and capabilities	One who has self-confidence: • Is confident in his or her job capability • Knows one's own strengths and believes in his or her own abilities • Displays a self-assurance that is visible to others • Has presence
SELF-MANAGEMENT	
Emotional self-control: Keeping disruptive emotions and impulses in check	One who has emotional self-control: • Does not act impulsively • Does not get impatient or show frustration • Behaves calmly in stressful situations • Stays composed and positive, even in trying moments

(continues)

Transparency: Maintaining integrity, acting congruently with one's values	One who exhibits transparency: • Keeps promises • Addresses unethical behavior in others • Openly and publicly admits to mistakes • Lives and acts on values
Adaptability: Flexibility in handling change	One who is adaptable: • Adapts ideas based on new information • Applies standard procedures flexibly • Handles unexpected demands well • Changes overall strategy, goals, or projects to fit the situation
Achievement: Striving to improve or meeting a standard of excellence	One who exhibits achievement: • Seeks ways to improve performance • Sets measurable and challenging goals • Anticipates obstacles to a goal • Takes calculated risks to reach a goal
Initiative: Readiness to act on opportunities	One who has initiative: • Does not hesitate to act on opportunities • Seeks information in unusual ways • Cuts through red tape and bends rules when necessary • Initiates actions to create possibilities
Optimism: Persistence in pursuing goals despite obstacles and setbacks	One who has optimism: • Has mainly positive expectations • Believes the future will be better than the past • Stays positive despite setbacks • Learns from setbacks
SOCIAL AWARENESS	
Empathy: Sensing others' feelings and perspectives and taking an active interest in their concerns	One who has empathy: • Listens attentively • Is attentive to people's moods or nonverbal cues • Relates well to people of diverse backgrounds • Can see things from someone else's perspective

(continues)

Organizational awareness: Reading a group's emotional currents and power relationships	One who has organizational awareness: • Is able to detect crucial social networks and key power relationships • Understands political forces within the organization • Identifies the organization's guiding values • Recognizes unspoken rules of the organization
Service: Anticipating, recognizing, and meeting customers' or clients' needs	One who provides service: • Makes himself available as needed • Monitors client satisfaction • Fosters an environment that keeps client relationships on the right track • Ensures that client needs are met
RELATIONSHIP MANAGEMENT	
Inspirational leadership: Inspiring and guiding individuals and groups	One who provides inspirational leadership: • Leads by example • Makes work exciting • Inspires others • Articulates a compelling vision
Influence: Having impact on others	• One who has influence: • Engages an audience when presenting • Persuades by appealing to people's self-interest • Gets support from key people • Develops behind-the-scenes support
Developing others: Sensing others' development needs and bolstering their abilities	One who develops others: • Recognizes specific strengths of others • Gives directions or demonstrations to develop someone • Gives constructive feedback • Provides ongoing mentoring or coaching
Change catalyst: Initiating or managing change.	One who is a change catalyst: • States need for change • Is not reluctant to change or make changes • Personally leads change initiatives • Advocates change despite opposition

Conflict management: Negotiating and resolving conflict.	One who manages conflict: • Airs disagreements or conflicts • Publicly states everyone's position to those involved in a conflict • Does not avoid conflict • Finds a position everyone can endorse
Teamwork and collaboration: Working with others and creating group synergy in pursuing collective goals.	One who exhibits teamwork and collaboration: • Cooperates with others • Solicits others' input • In a group, encourages others' participation • Establishes and maintains close relationships at work

Data from: Goleman, D., Boyatzis, R. and McKee, A. (2002). *Primal Leadership: Realizing the Power of Emotional Intelligence*. Boston, MA: Harvard Business School Press.

may lack the necessary emotional and relational competencies that enable them to lead and/or manage effectively (Goleman et al., 2002). They also need personal and social skills, which are the bases for emotional intelligence and are essential for effective leadership. In a team environment, skills such as effective listening, adaptability, empathy, collaboration, and the ability to give and use feedback are requisite for not only the designated leader, but for all members of the team. When members of a team are emotionally intelligent, they can create a collaborative atmosphere that leverages the inherent skills and power of the whole group (Goleman et al, 2002).

Resonance

The perceived attitude and emotional status of the leader is instrumental in the creation of a positive or negative emotional climate (Nembhard & Edmondson, 2006; Pescosolido, 2000). When a leader is impatient, frustrated, or fearful of failure, the group members react with defensive and self-protective behaviors—often setting off a reciprocal volley of destructive emotions and creating a dissonant and unproductive climate that is focused on self-preservation rather than cocreation. Conversely, leaders who project enthusiasm, realistic optimism, and care for the group engender these same feelings within the group. The group members are engaged, in sync, or are resonant with the leader and each other and have more energy to engage in the work of the group and face challenges more creatively (Pescosolido, 2000).

According to Boyatzis & McKee (2005), resonant leaders are mindful, compassionate, and hopeful and are skilled in eliciting affiliative and affirmative emotions in others. They are mindful in that they are fully aware of themselves, others, and the environment and are committed to their values while being open to other perspectives. The manifestation of hopefulness is confidence in their own and the group's ability to reify dreams. Compassion is reflected in their acceptance that they, in concert with their fellow humans, have strengths and vulnerabilities and are not omniscient. They face challenges and opportunities with equanimity and respect the contributions and value of the people they lead and those they serve.

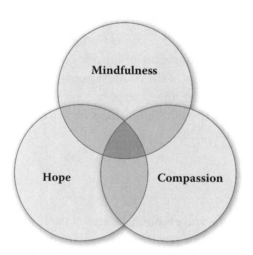

FIGURE 4-2 The resonant leader.

Data from: Boyatzis, R. & McKee, A. (2005). *Resonant Leadership.* Boston, MA: Harvard Business School Press.

There seems to be agreement that the best leaders are self-aware, self-regulating, and attuned to the diverse perspectives, needs, and abilities of their followers and the requirements of the situation. Good leaders have high levels of social and emotional intelligence, an ability to develop and maintain reciprocal relationships, and a willingness to empower others, and they are able to employ a balance of task-related and relation-building behaviors. Put simply, good leaders can get the job done well while maintaining a supportive emotional atmosphere (Goleman, 1998; Kouzes & Posner, 2007; Maxwell, 2005; Whitney et al, 2010).

References

Avolio, B. (2007). Promoting more integrative strategies for leadership theory building. *American Psychologist, 62,* 25–33.

Bass, B. M., & Avolio, B. J. (Eds.). (1994). *Improving organizational effectiveness through transformational leadership.* Thousand Oaks, CA: Sage Publications.

Blanchard, K., Zigarmi, P., & Zigarmi, D. (1985). *Leadership and the One Minute Manager.* New York: William Morrow.

Blake, R. & Mouton, J. (1978). *The new managerial grid.* Houston, TX: Gulf.

Blake, R. & Mouton, J. (1980). *The versatile manager: A Grid profile.* Homewood, IL: Dow Jones/Irwin.

Blake, R. & Mouton, J. (1982). How to choose a leadership style. *Training and Development Journal, 36,* 39–46.

Boyatzis, R., & McKee, A. (2005). *Resonant leadership.* Boston, MA: Harvard Business School Press.

Carlyle, T. (1841). *On heroes, hero worship and the heroic in history.* UK: James Fraser.

Fiedler, F. (1967). *A theory of leadership effectiveness.* New York, NY: McGraw-Hill.

Fiedler, F. (1978). The contingency model and the dynamics of the leadership process. *Advances in Experimental Social Psychology, 12,* 59–112.

Goleman, D. (1995). *Emotional intelligence.* New York, NY: Bantam Books.

Goleman, D. (1998). *Working with emotional intelligence.* New York, NY: Bantam Books.

Goleman, D., Boyatzis, R., & McKee, A. (2002). *Primal leadership: Learning to lead with emotional intelligence.* Boston, MA: Harvard Business School Press.

Goleman, D. & Boyatzis, R. (2008). Social intelligence and the biology of leadership. *Harvard Business Review, 89*(9), 74–81.

Hersey, P. (1985). *The situational leader.* New York, NY: Warner Books.

Hersey, P., & Blanchard, K. (1976). Leader effectiveness and adaptability description (LEAD). In J. W. Pfeiffer & J. E. Jones (Eds), *The 1976 annual handbook for group facilitators* (Vol. 5). La Jolla, CA: University Associates.

Hersey, P., & Blanchard, K. (1982). *Management of organizational behavior: Utilizing human resources* (4th ed.). Englewood Cliffs, NJ: Prentice Hall.

Jung, C. G. (1991). *The development of personality.* Collected Works Vol. 17. London, England: Routledge.

Kouzes, J. and Posner, B. (2007). *The leadership challenge.* San Franciso, CA: Jossey-Bass.

Maxwell, J. C. (2005). *The 360° leader: Developing your influence from anywhere in the organization.* Nashville, TN: Nelson Business.

McCrae, R., & Costa, P. (1987). Validation of the five factor model of personality across instruments and observers. *Journal of Personality and Social Psychology, 52*, 81–90.

Myers, I., McCaulley, M., Quenk, N. & Hammer, A.(1998). *MBTI Manual: A guide to the development and use of the Myers-Briggs Type Indicator*, 3rd edition. Mountainview, CA: Consulting Psychologists Press.

Nembhard, I., & Edmondson, A. (2006). Making it safe: The effects of leader inclusiveness and professional status on psychological safety and improvement efforts in health care teams. *Journal of Organizational Behavior, 27*, 941–966.

Northouse, P. (2010). *Leadership: Theory and practice.* Thousand Oaks, CA: SAGE Publications, Inc.

Pescosolido, A. T. (2000). *The leader's emotional impact in work groups* (Doctoral dissertation). Case Western Reserve University, Cleveland, OH.

Tolstoy, L. (1869). *War and peace.*

Whitney, D., Trosten-Bloom, A., & Radu, K. (2010). *Appreciative leadership: Focus on what works to drive winning performance.* New York, NY: McGraw Hill.

Zaccaro, S. (2007). Trait based perspectives of leadership. *American Psychologist, 62,* 6–16.

CHAPTER 5

Leadership Building Blocks

© AbleStock

Learning Objectives

1. Analyze the sources of power.
2. Understand the concept of cocreative power.
3. Analyze how motivation affects leadership styles.
4. Analyze how learning style affects leadership behaviors.
5. Understand the relationship of self-directed learning and personal transformation.

The most recent thinking on leadership recognizes an interaction between traits, styles, context and social dynamics. Good leaders can reflect on their behavior and evaluate their personal strengths, weaknesses, biases, needs and motivations. The honest appraisal of their own gifts and vulnerabilities engenders empathy for the gifts and vulnerabilities of others. This appreciation of the perspective of others facilitates a collaborative attitude that engages and inspires others to action.

The study of how leadership has evolved and the requisite knowledge, skills, and attitudes for effective leadership fall into the following three broad categories: power, motivation, and learning.

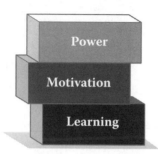

FIGURE 5-1   Power–motivation–learning.

Power

In the 1960s classic on management, *The Human Side of Enterprise*, Douglas McGregor examined the effects of leading/managing behaviors on subordinates using the theory X and theory Y approaches. In summary, theory X contends that employees are motivated mainly by money and must be controlled, directed, and threatened with punishment in order to work toward the achievement of organizational objectives. Theory Y, on the other hand, focuses on the creation of an environment that rewards the exercise of initiative, ingenuity, and self-direction and views opportunities for engagement and self-actualization as motivating forces. Leaders will often speak about their beliefs and philosophies of leadership as if they are aligned with theory Y. However, their actions are more reflective of theory X persuasion. Research has shown that inviting participation, facilitating positive friendly group and employee manager interaction, and giving workers responsibility improve productivity. However theory X informs many management decisions (Ryan & Deci, 2000; Spreier, Fontaine, & Malloy, 2006). The command and control aspect of theory X may frequently yield short-term results while sacrificing social capital, engagement, loyalty, and sustained productivity that is associated with theory Y (Spreitzer & Porath, 2012).

The exercise of authority is necessary in order for a group to form and for it to develop. In other words, someone needs to step up to the plate to get the ball rolling. However, in order for groups to mature, power and authority have to be distributed evenly over time. The distribution of authority and power in groups is as much a function of a person's position in the organization as it is the perception that group members have of that person. In the absence of specific information to the contrary, group members often attribute high or low status and related power and authority to individuals based on certain physical characteristics (height, strength), gender, race, ethnic or professional association (physician, professor, lawyer) (Berger, Cohen, & Zeldich, 1972). French and Raven (1959) defined four catagories of power. Referent power means that power is inferred by means of status or personal characteristics such as charm or decisiveness. In other words, people make an assumption that a person who is a physician will be a leader since being a physician is considered a high-status position. Legitimate power resides with the person, such as a CEO, who by nature of his/her position, wields power. Expert power belongs to those who have specialized knowledge, information, and skills. Coercive power relates to the ability to distribute positive/negative reinforcers.

Power and status differentials are a fact of life and frequently limit the participation of team members who perceive themselves to be of lower status. Limitations in participation are often related to reduced engagement in the group process along with diminished accountability for group outcomes. If this disengagement is experienced by the members of a team who do not hold high-status positions, the team will not benefit from their expertise, and the team will not have the cohesion necessary to reach its functional potential. Leaders can mitigate the effects of status and

REFLECTION: *Who's Got the Power?*

If a CEO, a physician, and a sailor were on a storm-tossed ship, who do you think would be the most powerful of the three? What kind of power does he/she have?

Suppose the CEO, physician, and sailor land safely on a remote island that houses a secret military base. They are mistaken for spies and taken to the base commander who will determine their fate. Describe how the commander might exercise coercive power.

power differentials on group participation by making a conscious effort to create a psychologically safe atmosphere where inclusive participation is the norm (Nembhard & Edmondson, 2006). The literature is replete with examples of how the traditional hierarchies in healthcare practices have proved detrimental to the harnessing of the power of the collective intelligence that exists among diverse groups of healthcare workers (Drinka & Clarke, 2000; Freshman, Rubino, & Chassiako, 2010; Garman, Leach & Spector, 2006; Gittell, 2009; Gray, 2008; IOM, 2001, 2003; Lee, 2010). Recent research suggests that in groups without a designated leader, power is given in the form of attention to the individuals who are the most emotionally expressive and who have the most valued traits (Goleman, 2011). These assumptions, in combination with the traditional medical hierarchy and actual differences in disciplinary cultures, professional education, experience, and responsibility, contribute to the variations in dominance, prestige, and control in healthcare teams.

> *Power over* is a traditional relationship in which one person has power over another person or one group over another group . . . It is a relationship of polarity. *Power with* is at once relational and collective . . . an organizational form of collaboration . . . *cocreative power*. Power with has the boldness to believe that acting from immediate self interest is not always the wisest course of action, nor that one person or one group should be in a position to know what is best for the other . . . (Briskin, Erickson, Ott, & Callanan, 2009, p. 94)

There is another orientation that reflects the interconnectedness that is characteristic of Eastern traditions. *Cocreative power* is a term that was coined by Mary Parker Follett early in the twentieth century. Her ideas reflected systems theory and the integrative, reflective practices that are considered hallmarks of learning organizations, successful agents of change, and innovative groups. These notions continued to resonate and informed the emergence of concepts such as participatory management, quality circles, and team-based approaches to distributed leadership in groups (Briskin et al., 2009).

REFLECTION: *Power Assessment*

Identify two individuals who you think are powerful.

List the specific behaviors each of them uses in exercising that power.

What type of power are they using?

Is one individual more effective than the other? Why?

Could you see yourself using power in the same way?

Why? Why not?

Motivation

David McClelland (1953, 1987) hypothesized that human behavior is a result of a complex mix of motivations—some of which are stronger than others. McClelland found that most behavior can be related to three social motives or needs. These needs are achievement, affiliation, and power. Achievement motive describes the drive to attain challenging goals and exceed expected results. People with a high need for achievement revel in accomplishing something no one has done before. High-achievers want jobs where they can succeed based on their expertise. For managers in large organizations, moderate to high achievement is secondary to higher power needs. If achievement is dominant, a manager may try to achieve objectives alone rather than through team development (Yukl, 1989). Affiliation motive describes the need for friendly and close relationships. People with high affiliation tend to like to work with others and value harmony and collaboration. People with a high affiliation motive tend to value harmonious relationships and will do whatever they can in the workplace to preserve relationships. Power motive describes the need to control or strongly influence another person or group's behavior. There is a strong need to lead and for their ideas to prevail. There is also motivation and need toward increasing personal status and prestige.

Power motive is often misunderstood as a negative trait. Yukl (1989) differentiates between personal power and socialized power. People with highly personalized power may have little inhibition or self-control, and they exercise power impulsively. When they give advice or support, it is with strategic intent to further bolster their own status. They demand loyalty to their leadership rather than to the organization. When the leader leaves the organization there is likely disorder and breakdown of team morale and direction. Socialized power need is most often associated with effective leadership. These leaders direct their power in socially positive ways that benefit others and the organization rather than only contributing to the leader's status and gain. They seek power because it is through power that tasks are accomplished. They recognize that power must be distributed and shared and that other people need to have power over their own work lives. Effective leaders empower others who use that power to enact and further the leader's vision for the organization.

McClelland (1953, 1987) hypothesized that the most successful leaders appear to be driven mainly by the need to achieve, in combination with a need to empower others and forge relationships. Further research yielded that primary motivating factors informed specific leadership behavioral styles, such as directive, pace setting, visionary, affiliative, participative, and coaching styles. Exclusive use of any one style can lead to unintended, negative consequences. For instance, highly directive and pacesetting leaders may micromanage and focus on goals rather than people, which can lead to demoralized and disengaged teams. However, leaders who are myopic in their attention to relationship building may avoid giving negative feedback, avoid confrontation, and worry so much about people that they lose their ability to objectively evaluate performance. Leaders who had a repertoire of visionary, affiliative, participative, and coaching behaviors created energizing work climates but those who were primarily pacesetting tended to create neutral or demotivating work climates. The most effective leaders are those who have a curiosity and respect for their own and others' needs, motivation, strengths and weaknesses, and preferred modes of learning, as well as an ability to adjust their style and structure the situation so that they are complementary and facilitate positive outcomes (Spreier et al., 2006).

A tool that is often used for self-discovery and leadership development is the Fundamental Interpersonal Relations Orientation (FIRO) (Schutz, 1958). The FIRO is based on the theory that there are three primary motivating factors for individuals' behavior in groups. These factors are inclusion, control, and affection. For example, people who are motivated primarily by the need for inclusion will tend to be very social and interactive. Those who are driven by the need to control might be autocratic in their dealings with others, while those who have a strong desire to be liked may spend a great deal of time developing strong relationships.

Measurements from the FIRO and the Myers-Briggs Type Indicators are highly correlated and are often used together to provide a typology for assessing the primary motivating factors for leaders' behaviors and the preferred behavioral style associated with those needs. These assessments are used for self-discovery and learning and are not designed to be used for evaluative purposes.

TABLE 5-1 Leadership Style Summary

Leadership Style	Focus	Purpose
Directive	Moving toward immediate action. Gives clear directions	Decisive action in emergency situations
Visionary	Clear communication. Move people toward shared dreams	Provide redirection for change initiatives
Affiliative	Harmonious relationships	Bridge building and motivation during stressful times
Participative	Consensus building, engagement and commitment	Developing collective buy-in
Pacesetting	Meeting challenges	Achieving high quality results with highly competent team
Coaching	Development and mentoring of others	Building longterm team and organizational capabilities

Data from: Spreier, S., Fontaine, M. and Malloy, R. (2006, June) Leadership run amok: The destructive potential of overachievers. *Harvard Business Review*, 73–82.

It is understood that power can arise from an individual's personal characteristics or social status (referent power), position (legitimate power), specialized skill (expert power), or ability to distribute rewards or punishment (coercive power) (French & Raven, 1959). There are some individuals who possess all four sources of power by virtue of their status and personal magnetism, their designated position in the organization, their expertise, and their ability to dispense rewards and punishment. Does this make them influential and effective leaders? You would have to examine how the person exercised power and what effect it had on the followers before you could judge his or her success as a leader. How transformational and sustainable was his or her effect on others' behavior? Did the followers merely do as they were told or did they internalize the leader's message and move forward inspired by a mission?

Learning

Self-awareness and the ability to consider the impact of interactive and learning styles on group function and to change accordingly are hallmarks of transformational learning and effective leadership (Goleman, 1995; Hersey & Blanchard, 1976, 1982; Whitney, Trosten-Bloom, & Radu, 2010). Successful healthcare team leaders and members must navigate multiple relationships, be open to new ideas, solve complex problems, and generate innovative and effective solutions. Adjusting, adapting, and innovating are all, in essence, outcomes of learning (Brown & Posner, 2001; Vaill, 1998). Leadership is a developmental process that can be viewed as a lifelong journey that incorporates the cognitive (what you learn) and metacognitive (how you learn) aspects of learning. An understanding of adult learning theories and their relationship to the development of leadership behaviors will help healthcare team members to adapt and thrive in complex healthcare environments.

Andragogy—the study of adult learning—posits that over time, humans develop fixed ideas—cognitive structures or fixed gestalts regarding themselves and the world around them. Learning happens when an individual's established ideas are challenged through experience or conflicting external forces (Knowles, Holton, & Swanson, 2005). The literature regarding learning and leadership corroborates andragogy's premise. Leaders tend to learn best when learning is self-directed, transformational, and experiential (Brown & Posner, 2001; Dalton, 1999; Kouzes & Posner, 2007; Mirriam, Caffarella & Baumgartner, 2007; Zemke, 1985).

Self-directed learning means that adult learners need to be autonomous in what they learn, when they learn, and how they learn. Adults must be given enough information and background to understand why they should take the time to learn something new. Learning activities must be interactive, adaptable to differing learning styles, and applicable to real life situations.

Mezirow (1981) identified an individual's overall worldview as "meaning perspective" that is generated in childhood and composed of values, beliefs, and experiences. Meaning perspectives serve as perceptual filters and determine how an individual will organize and interpret the meaning of his/her life's experiences. When schemas are disrupted by new experiences, information, traumatic life events, ideas, or concepts, transformational learning takes place and alter our view on the micro and macro level (Clarke, 1993; Mezirow, 1981; Mirriam et al., 2007). Inherent to this perceptual shift is the realization that individuals can explore new behaviors and liberate their power as agents of change rather than victims of change. This personal transformation increases self-efficacy and the confidence to employ leadership behaviors to impact not only personal growth but change and growth in the people and groups outside of oneself (Friere, 1973).

Adults learn best when they can engage in experiential learning and employ the wisdom of past experiences when meeting new challenges. Leaders will almost always cite trial and error experiences rather than formal coursework as their most pivotal learning events (Bryan, 2011).

Kolb (1974) developed a cyclical model of adult learning that includes concrete experiences, reflective observations, abstract conceptualizations, and active experimentation. The most valuable adult learning experiences are characterized by opportunities to act, reflect on the action, obtain feedback on the action,

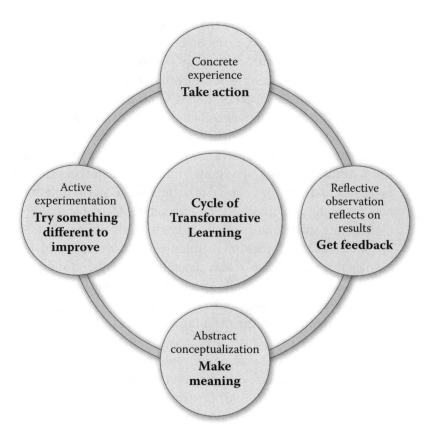

FIGURE 5-2 Kolb model of adult learning.

Adapted from: Kolb, D. (1974). On management and the learning process. In D. Kolb, I. Rubin, & J. McIntyre (Eds.), Organizational psychology: A book of readings (pp. 27–42). Englewood Cliffs, NJ: Prentice Hall.

make sense of the experience, and engage in active experimentation of alternative actions.

The Kolb Learning Style Inventory (LSI) (1974) is a self-report questionnaire that yields scores in the following four learning modes: concrete experience (CE), reflective observation (RO), abstract conceptualization (AC), and active experimentation (AE).

Convergers have high scores in the AC and AE areas and like to engage in the practical application of theories to solve specific

TABLE 5-2   Kolb Learning Modes Summary

Concrete Experience (CE)	Learns by direct experience, discussion, and feedback from others
Reflective Observation (RO)	Learns by listening and reflecting
Abstract Conceptualization (AC)	Learns by logical thinking and objective analysis
Active Experimentation (AE)	Learns by active engagement

Adapted from: Kolb, D. (1974). On management and the learning process. In D. Kolb, I. Rubin, & J. McIntyre (Eds.), *Organizational psychology: A book of readings* (pp. 27–42). Englewood Cliffs, NJ: Prentice Hall.

problems. Divergers have high scores in CE and RO. They are imaginative and creative and like to see situations from many perspectives. Assimilators score highest in the AC and RO areas and excel in developing theoretical concepts. Accommodators score highest in the CE and AE areas and prefer risk taking and solving problems in a collaborative, trial-and-error fashion.

In addition to tools such as the FIRO, MBTI—measurements such as the Kolb Learning Inventory serve to further expand self-knowledge. In short, the Kolb inventory provides a method for understanding whether one learns best by trial and error, developing theory, applying theory to practice, or collaborating with others. In addition to broadening a potential leader's self-knowledge, these tools also serve as a point of reference when trying to comprehend and influence the behavior of others. A leader has a much better chance of understanding and influencing others when he/she takes the time to address their interests and perspectives.

REFLECTION: *Kolb Learning Styles Summary*

Review the summary of the Kolb learning styles in Table 5-3. Which style best describes you? What impact does your preferred learning style have on your emerging leadership?

TABLE 5-3 Kolb Learning Styles

Accommodating Style	Diverging Style
Focusing on the vision and strategy for the future energizes this type of learner. This type of learner:	*Focusing on values and leadership energizes this type of learner. This type of learner:*
• Thrives on crisis and challenge • Looks for patterns to solve problems • Leads by energizing people • Influences through holding up a positive vision of the future • Works hard to win—making sure the organization is a front runner • Needs a staff that can follow up and implement details	• Thrives on taking time to develop good ideas • Tackles problems through brainstorming with staff • Leads by the heart • Involves others in decision making • Influences through trust and participation • Works for organizational solidarity • Needs a staff that is supportive and shares sense of mission or vision
Converging Style	**Assimilating Style**
Focusing on getting things done to improve quality energizes this type of learner. This type of learner:	*Focusing on the facts and developing new theories and models energizes this type of learner. This type of learner:*
• Thrives on plans and project management • Tackles problems by making unilateral decisions • Leads by personal forcefulness • Values and inspires quality • Influences through rewards and punishment • Creates efficient rules and enforces them • Works hard for organizational efficiency and solvency • Needs task-oriented staff to move quickly	• Thrives on assimilating disparate facts into coherent theories • Tackles problems with rationality and logic • Leads by principles • Follows rules and processes • Influences through persuasion and facts in order to get things done • Works to enhance the organizations as an embodiment of tradition and prestige • Needs staff members who are well organized, write things on paper, and follow through on agreed-upon decisions

Adapted from: Kolb, D. (1974). On management and the learning process. In D. Kolb, I. Rubin, & J. McIntyre (Eds.), *Organizational psychology: A book of readings* (pp. 27–42). Englewood Cliffs, NJ: Prentice Hall.

REFLECTION: *Self-Management—
Mature Leader Reflection*

At the heart of self-management lies an ability to reflect on one's own behavior, values, and style and the effect they have on others and the effect other peoples' values, behaviors, and styles have on oneself.
Mature leaders learn to:

1. Stretch beyond their own personal learning style so that they can learn in every situation, even if it is not designed for their personal preference.

2. Be conscious of other people's preferred style and adjust communication accordingly.

Answer the following questions:

1. What does your style tell you about what you are really good at?

2. How would learning to act and work with those with opposite preferences help you be seen as a leader by others?

References

Bryan, A. (2011). *The corner office: Indispensable and unexpected lessons from CEOs on how to lead and succeed.* New York, NY: Times Books/Henry Holt & Co.

Clarke, M. (1993). Transformational learning. *New directions for adults and continuing education, 57,* 47–56.

Dalton, M. (1999). *The learning tactics inventory.* San Francisco, CA: Jossey-Bass/Pfieffer.

Drinka, T., & Clark, P. (2000). *Health care teamwork: Interdisciplinary practice and teaching.* Westport, CT: Auburn House.

French, J., & Raven, B. (1959). The bases of social power. In D. Cartwright & A. Zander. *Group dynamics* (pp. 259–269). New York, NY: Harper & Row.

Freshman, B., Rubino, L., & Chassiako, Y. (2010). *Collaboration across the disciplines in health care.* Sudbury, MA: Jones and Bartlett.

Friere, P. (1973). *Pedagogy of the oppressed.* New York, NY: Seabury Press.

Garman, A., Leach, D., & Spector, N. (2006). Worldviews in collision: Conflict and collaboration across professional lines. *Journal of Organizational Behaviour, 27,* 829–849.

Gittell, J. (2009). *High performance healthcare: Using the power of relationships to achieve quality, efficiency and resilience.* New York, NY: McGraw-Hill.

Goleman, D. (1995). *Emotional intelligence.* New York, NY: Bantam Books.

Goleman, D. (1998). *Working with emotional intelligence.* New York, NY: Bantam Books.

Goleman, D. (2003). *Destructive emotions: A scientific dialogue with the Dalai Lama.* New York, NY: Bantam Books.

Goleman, D. (2011). *Leadership: The power of emotional intelligence.* Northampton, MA: More Than Sound.

Gray, B. (2008). Enhancing transdisciplinary research through collaborative leadership. *American Journal of Preventive Medicine, 35*(2S), s124–s132.

Hersey, P., & Blanchard, K. (1976). Leader effectiveness and adaptability description (LEAD). In J. W. Pfeiffer & J. E. Jones (Eds). *The 1976 annual handbook for group facilitators* (Vol. 5). La Jolla, CA: University Associates.

Hersey, P., & Blanchard, K. (1982). *Management of organizational behavior: Utilizing human resources* (4th ed.). Englewood Cliffs, NJ: Prentice Hall.

Institutes of Medicine. (2001). *Crossing the quality chasm: A new health system for the 21st century.* Washington, DC: National Academy Press.

Institutes of Medicine. (2002). *Who will keep the public healthy? Educating public health professionals for the 21st century.* Washington, DC: National Academy Press.

Institutes of Medicine. (2003). *Health professions education: A bridge to quality.* Washington, DC: National Academy Press.

Knowles, M., Holton, E., & Swanson, R. (2005). *The adult learner: The definitive classic in adult education and human resource development* (6th ed.). Burlington, MA: Elsevier.

Kolb, D. (1974). On management and the learning process. In D. Kolb, I. Rubin, & J. McIntyre (Eds.), *Organizational psychology: A book of readings* (pp. 27–42). Englewood Cliffs, NJ: Prentice Hall.

Kouzes, J., & Posner, B. (2007). *The leadership challenge.* San Francisco, CA: Jossey-Bass.

Lee, T. (2010, April). Turning doctors into leaders. *Harvard Business Review*, pp. 50–58.

McClelland, D. (1953). *The achievement motive.* New York, NY: Appleton-Century Crofts.

McClelland, D. (1987). *Human motivation.* Cambridge, UK: Cambridge University Press.

Mezirow, J. (1981). A critical theory of adult learning and education. *Adult Education Quarterly, 32*(1), 3–24.

Mirriam, S., Caffarella, R., & Baumgartner, L. (2007). *Learning in adulthood: A comprehensive guide.* San Francisco, CA: Jossey-Bass.

Nembhard, I., & Edmondson, A. (2006). Making it safe: The effects of leader inclusiveness and professional status on psychological safety and improvement efforts in health care teams. *Journal of Organizational Behavior, 27*, 941–966.

Ryan, R., & Deci, E. (2000). Self determination theory and the facilitation of intrinsic motivation, social development and well being. *American Psychologist, 55*, 68–78.

Schutz, W. (1958). *FIRO: A three dimensional theory of interpersonal behavior.* New York, NY: Rienhart.

Spreier, S., Fontaine, M., & Malloy, R. (2006, June). Leadership run amok: The destructive potential of overachievers. *Harvard Business Review*, 73–82.

Spreitzer, G., & Porath, C. (2012, January–February). Creating sustainable performance. *Harvard Business Review, 90*(1–2), 92–99.

Vaill, P. (1998). *Spirited leading and learning.* San Francisco, CA: Jossey-Bass.

Whitney, D., Trosten-Bloom, A., & Radu, K. (2010). *Appreciative leadership: Focus on what works to drive winning performance.* New York, NY: McGraw-Hill.

Yukl, G. A. (1989). *Leadership in organizations.* Englewood Cliffs, NJ: Prentice Hall.

Zemke, R. (1985) The Honeywell studies: How managers learn to manage. *Training, 22*(8), 46–51.

CHAPTER 6

Relational Leadership

Learning Objectives

1. Demonstrate self-awareness, self-understanding, respect, empathy, altruism, and self-disclosure through participation in groups.
2. Identify a personal leadership style and construct a personal philosophy of leadership.
3. Explain the various attitudes and roles that an effective leader must assume.
4. Evaluate the effect of personal leadership behaviors on oneself and other members of the team.
5. Use reflection and inquiry to facilitate personal and group development.

Members of the healthcare professions are well schooled in the aspects of mindfulness, hope, and compassion—as they apply to their relationships with their patients. Compassion and empathy for others are often the motivation for pursuing a healthcare career. Good clinical reasoning requires focused examination of objective clinical information in combination with mindful, in-the-moment analysis of the unique, subjective illness experience of each patient. Hope—the firm belief in the capability of the health professions and the resilience of the human spirit to overcome adversity and positively affect the quality of patients' lives—lies at the very core of every health profession. The challenge for leaders and members of healthcare teams is to understand that it is their responsibility to take a leadership stance and employ these qualities not only with their patients but also in their interactions with coworkers, superiors, and subordinates.

Zolno (2007) perceives leadership as a relational act that is facilitated by a personal sense of self-worth, hope, and capability. Individuals who develop their own sense of worth, hopes, and capabilities can, through the building of positive relationships, transmit those values to others. Zolno and Skillman (2011) further describe leadership as a multifaceted action that is generative, affirmative, collaborative, catalytic, and harmonizing (see **Table 6-1**). Each of these terms address the relational nature of

TABLE 6-1 Multifaceted Leadership as Described by Zolno and Skillman

Attitude	Role	Skill
Generative	Learner	Comfortable with not knowing Openness to new learning Ability to learn from experience and apply knowledge to new situations Solicit feedback from all constituencies
Affirmative	Coach	• Ability to focus on strengths, successes, positive intentions, and potential of others • Ability to broaden the perceptions of others in order to formulate new behavioral choices
Collaborative	Partner	• Create an inclusive atmosphere where all ideas are welcomed and valued
Catalytic	Catalyst	• Leverage diversity of thought • Encourage exploration outside the box • Challenge the status quo
Harmonizing	Ecologist	• Ability to understand and capitalize on the interactive and interdependent nature of social systems

Data from: Zolno, S., Skillman, R. (2011). *Coaching Certification in Whole System IQ and Appreciative Inquiry.* Vaushon, WA: The Leading Clinic.

leadership and provides a framework for examining the roles that leaders must assume in order to become agents of positive change and growth in oneself and others.

The Leader as Learner

The highly specialized training that is the hallmark of traditional health professional education places a premium on knowing and leaves little room for understanding the perspectives of multiple disciplines. Those professionals who have a negative capability or an ability to not know are more comfortable working in the ambiguous space between disciplines and are more likely to

---

CASE STORY: *I Don't Know What You Are Talking About*

We need to have a more robust acknowledgment about the fact that we don't know how to run an interdisciplinary/interprofessional team. We pretend we all know how it works. We are embarrassed that we don't know how to do it. I don't know that people even know what interprofessional team-work means.

I noticed that when teams were meeting and people gave their perspective, they were using short hand. If you were in another discipline you didn't know what they were saying. As a nurse, I didn't understand what the occupational therapist was saying and the social worker didn't know what the nurse was saying. Everyone nodded their heads though, thinking that they were supposed to understand. It was like we are back in grade school and we don't want to admit that we don't know. After the meeting, people would confide in me that "I really had no idea what so and so was saying." I started to send a message in the organization that you should assume no one knows what you are talking about unless they are in your discipline. I started to help people recognize that we cannot use shorthand language in interdisciplinary teams. I suggested that people create a template for their own short hand and be more aware that everyone doesn't understand it and be willing to say "I don't know what you are talking about" if they don't know what someone is talking about.

—Kevin Hook, Chief Nursing Officer, University of Pennsylvania LIFE (Living Independently for Elders) Program

---

REFLECTION: *Lifelong Learning*

Leader and Members as Lifelong Learners	
Who do I want to be?	
Who am I now?	
How will I use my strengths to achieve my goals?	
Who will help me to achieve my goals?	

encourage innovative thought and creative solutions to complex problems (Hammick, et al, 2009; Whitney, Trosten-Bloom, & Radu, 2010). Leaders who attain a comfort level with "the tension inherent in not knowing" encourage all the members of their teams to question the status quo, think creatively, and seek new ways to approach problem solving (French, Harvey, & Sampson, 2001, p.7).

The Leader as Coach

Coaching can be defined as the building of deep relationships in order to equip people with the knowledge, skills and attitudes that will help them achieve their potential. (Peterson & Hicks, 1996). By increasing the self-efficacy of others, the coaching leader helps to broaden their perceived range of choices and possibilities for action. The core of the coaching process is informed by andragogy or adult learning theory, which assumes that the most meaningful learning experiences for adults are experiential, self-directed, and personally relevant (Knowles, Holton, & Swanson, 2005).

Kolb (1974) described adult learning as a cycle that includes concrete experiences, reflective observations, abstract conceptualizations, and active experimentation. In a coaching environment, a person is encouraged to attend to how they feel about an action, reflect on that experience, make sense out of the experience, and then explore a better way to take action next time.

The designated leader of the team actively coaches team members by learning to listen, learning to ask powerful questions and creating a safe environment based on trust and confidentiality. The leader of healthcare teams has a unique challenge in that he/she must be able to navigate between the traditional expert/novice model—"the sage on the stage"—of supervision/teaching, which requires the transmission of professional expertise and the "guide on the side" ability to engage others in active self-exploration and growth (McKee, Tilin, & Mason, 2009). A successful coaching relationship will create an atmosphere of respect and trust that will enable team members to assume a leadership stance and will allow them to offer their unique professional perspective while maintaining an active curiosity and actively soliciting the same from other team members. It has been suggested that coaching with compassion—helping others achieve their goals—triggers parasympathetic activity and actually counteracts the physiological and psychological effects of stress associated with positions of power (Boyatzis, Smith, & Blaize, 2006).

EXAMPLE *of a Leader as Coach*

A case manager has been experiencing difficulty getting her team to work together efficiently. She comes to her weekly session with her supervisor to discuss how she should handle this challenge. Her supervisor assumes a coaching stance and responds to the case manager's concerns:

- Can you tell me about interdisciplinary teams that have been really successful? (Concrete experience)
- Why were they successful? (Abstract conceptualization)
- What did you do to make the team successful? (Reflective observation)
- What did the members do? (Reflective observation)
- What can you do to make it more effective? (Active experimentation)

The Leader as Partner

A psychologically safe work environment mitigates the risk associated with behaviors that bridge status differentials such as suggesting new procedures, offering unsolicited feedback or sharing innovative ideas. Senior team members (those who hold high status positions as well as those who have been on the job longest) have a unique opportunity to enculturate new team members by modeling relationship-building behaviors that facilitate interpersonal trust, respect, and active engagement in collaborative team efforts. As the tenure of team members within a position increases, so does their communication and tendency to pay less attention to status differentials. As status barriers fade and team-wide collaboration increases, opportunities for creative problem solving and innovation abound. A key component of leadership development initiatives is learning how to be inclusive and to foster psychological safety within healthcare teams because this is linked to quality improvement in patient care (Nembhard & Edmondson, 2006).

The Leader as Catalyst

The focus on building relationships in order to empower others to act rather than the exercise of control over the actions of others is synonymous with the concept of servant leadership and particularly cogent to teams of health professionals. Servant leaders appreciate and leverage the expertise and contributions of every member of the healthcare team in order to enhance patient outcomes (Hammick et al, 2009; Neill, Hayward, & Peterson, 2007). Knowing when to defer to the expertise of others is a valuable trait for leaders/members of interdisciplinary healthcare teams. The strength of the team lies in its ability to leverage the skills of multiple disciplines toward the common goal of client-centered care. While individual members of the interdisciplinary team have a comfort level with traditionally prescribed roles and responsibilities, they must be cognizant of the limits of their knowledge and capabilities and reach beyond disciplinary boundaries in order to facilitate relationships and client-centered versus disciplinary-centered practice.

The Leader as Ecologist

With specialized training comes greater natural resistance to alternative methods and approaches as well as greater difficulty communicating approaches to others who are not similarly trained. Bridging the gaps between the disciplines is often a key role that healthcare leaders play for their organization (Garman, 2010). By deep listening—refocusing our attention on the orientation of others—instead of talking and by asking questions rather than making statements, leaders/members of healthcare teams can transform disciplinary boundaries from spaces of conflict to spaces of new learning and innovation in relationship-based, patient-centered care (French et al., 2001; Gray, 2008; Klein, 2010).

It appears that the most effective leaders are those whose allegiance to group goals supersedes personal goals or who have a strong other orientation. Gray (2008) suggests that leadership behaviors in well-functioning interdisciplinary groups can be demonstrated through cognitive, structural, and procedural tasks. Cognitive tasks often take the form of appreciative forms of inquiry where the focus is placed on how the team can make best practice the norm rather than how the team can avoid mistakes. Establishing strong social networks within the team and with stakeholders outside of the team are structural or bridge-building behaviors that serve to neutralize power and disciplinary differentials and garner universal engagement of all team members. Procedural tasks such as the design of meetings, the establishment of standards for information exchange, and conflict management insure constructive and productive decision making, innovative problem solving, and conflict resolution among team members.

The focus on building relationships in order to empower others to act rather than exercising control over the actions of others is synonymous with the concept of servant leadership and particularly cogent to teams of health professionals. Servant

CASE STORY: FINDING BALANCE

Sometimes we get bogged down in the discussion phase rather than the decision phase. Too much input makes things more complicated and time consuming. We work very closely together and sometimes the social life of the team overtakes the more evidence-based work aspects. We call ourselves a "family." A discussion about a problem with a member can devolve into a gossip session. The whole conversation deteriorates and rather than using data and evidence, our feelings, beliefs, and concepts get interwoven and we end up without a decision. We need to strike a balance between working with each other as a team and being a "family." What I do when this happens is refocus the team concentration. I say, "Hold it—Stop—Time out. That is fascinating, but here are the ideas on the table. What is the solution?" People appreciate the focusing.

—Karen J. Nichols, MD, Chief Medical Officer, The Life Practice, School of Nursing University of Pennsylvania Life Program

leaders appreciate and leverage the expertise and contributions of every member of the healthcare team in order to enhance patient outcomes (Hammick et al 2009; Neill, Hayward, & Peterson, 2007). Whitney, Trosten-Bloom and Radu (2010) maintain that the leader's primary responsibility in any group is to help others to recognize their strengths and value to the organization through inquiry, inclusion, illumination, and inspiration. Inquiry addresses the aspect of ongoing dialogue regarding best practices and opportunities for positive growth. Inclusion addresses the aspect of creating a psychologically safe environment where all voices are welcomed and heard. Illumination is addressed through the use of appreciative practices, which highlight exemplary performance such as success stories shared via newsletters or at the opening of each team meeting. Inspiration is addressed by modeling leadership behaviors and by providing opportunities for positive change and growth by 360-degree feedback in performance reviews and aligning job assignments with strengths and interests.

REFLECTION: *Leadership Development*

"The longest journey of any person is the journey inward." —Dag Hammarskjöld

Reflection is the process of changing one's perspective as new information and experiences are encountered. Leadership development is based, in part, on the ability to reflect on your own behavior and the effect it has on the behavior of others.

Think of a time that you assumed a leadership role in a group.

- Why do you think you assumed this role?
- What do you recall about your own behavior when you assumed this role?
- How did you feel when you assumed this role?
- How did others in the group respond to your assumption of this role?
- How did others in the group feel about your assumption of this role?
- How did you know what they felt?
- What was the outcome?
- Did the outcome surprise you? Why or why not?
- What might you have done differently?

Much of the early literature addressed leadership with a capital *L*. It dealt with specific traits or situations that distinguished one person from the crowd, attracted followers, and inspired great accomplishments that were products of the leader's singular vision. Current literature conceptualizes leadership—with a lowercase *l*—as a constellation of behaviors that helps others recognize their strengths, articulate their ideas, and engage in collaboration with others in order to achieve optimum results. Although the leadership competency models described by Garman (2010) were formulated for healthcare administrators, the overarching themes of communication and self-management resonate for all members of the healthcare team no matter what their position in the system hierarchy. Put simply, self-management entails attention to process and people in the form of structuring the work environment and developing work relationships.

High-level administrative turnover in the volatile healthcare industry highlights the importance of front-line healthcare workers assuming the leadership stance and becoming proactive in the creation and maintenance of resonant team cultures. Rather than *Leadership* being reserved for the few, *leadership behaviors* are viewed as requirements for all members of high-functioning healthcare teams. When leadership behaviors are the expected and respected norm of a group, traditional hierarchies break down, and active listening, knowledge sharing, collaborating, coaching, and continuous learning bridge the disciplines and enable the team members to achieve strong, sustainable relationships and provide exemplary patient-centered care (Becker-Reems & Garrett, 1998; Gittell, 2009).

References

Anchor, S. (2012, January–February). Positive intelligence. *Harvard Business Review, 90* (1–2). 100–102.

Becker-Reems, E., & Garrett, D. (1998). *Testing the limits of teams: How to implement self management in health care.* Chicago, IL: American Hospital Publishing, Inc.

Boyatzis, R., Smith, M., & Blaize, N. (2006). Developing sustainable leaders through coaching and compassion. *Academy of Management Learning & Education, 5*(1), 8–24.

Briskin, A., Erickson, S., Ott, J., & Callanan, T. (2009). *The power of collective wisdom and the trap of collective folly.* San Francisco, CA: Berrett-Koehler.

Fox, J. (2012, January–February). The economics of well being. *Harvard Business Review, 90* (1–2), 79–83.

French, R., Harvey, C., & Sampson, P. (June, 2001). *Negative capability: The key to creative leadership.* Presented at the International Society for the Psychoanalytic Study of Organizations symposia, Paris, France.

Garman, A. (2010). Leadership development in the interdisciplinary context. In B. Freshman, L. Rubino, & Y. Chassiakos (Eds.), *Collaboration across the disciplines in health care* (pp. 43–64). Sudbury, MA: Jones and Bartlett Learning.

Gittell, J. (2009). *High performance healthcare: Using the power of relationships to achieve quality, efficiency and resilience.* New York, NY: McGraw-Hill.

Gray, B. (2008). Enhancing transdisciplinary research through collaborative leadership. *American Journal of Preventive Medicine, 35*(2S), s124–s132.

Hammick, M., Freeth, D., Copperman, J., & Goodsman, D. (2009). *Being interprofessional.* Malden, MA: Polity Press.

Institutes of Medicine, Committee on Quality of Health Care in America, National Academy of Sciences. (2001). *Crossing the Quality Chasm: A new health system for the 21st Century.* Washington, DC: National Academy Press.

Institutes of Medicine, Committee on Quality of Health Care in America, National Academy of Sciences. (2002). *Who will keep the public healthy? Educating public health professionals for the 21st century.* Washington, DC: National Academy Press.

Institutes of Medicine, Committee on Quality of Health Care in America, National Academy of Sciences. (2003). *Health Professions Education: A bridge to quality.* Washington, DC: National Academy Press.

Institutes of Medicine. (2002). *Who will keep the public healthy? Educating public health*

Klein, J. (2010). *Creating interdisciplinary campus cultures: A model for strength and sustainability.* San Francisco, CA: Jossey-Bass.

Knowles, M., Holton, E., & Swanson, R. (2005). *The adult learner: The definitive classic in adult education and human resource development* (6th ed.). Burlington, MA: Elsevier.

Kolb, D. (1974). On management and the learning process. In D. Kolb, I. Rubin, & J. McIntyre (Eds.), *Organizational psychology: A book of readings* (pp. 27–42). Englewood Cliffs, NJ: Prentice Hall.

McKee, A., Tilin, F., & Mason, D. (2009). Coaching from the inside: Building an internal group of emotionally intelligent coaches. *International Coaching Psychology Review, 4*(1), 35–46.

Neill, M., Hayward, K. S., & Peterson, T. (2007). Students' perceptions of the interprofessional team in practice through the application of servant leadership principles. *Journal of Inter-professional Care, 21*(4), 425–432.

Nembhard, I., & Edmondson, A. (2006). Making it safe: The effects of leader inclusiveness and professional status on psychological safety and improvement efforts in health care teams. *Journal of Organizational Behavior, 27,* 941–966.

Peterson, D. & Hicks, M (1996). *Leader as coach: Strategies for coaching and developing others.* Minneapolis, MN: Personnel Decisions International.

Pew Health Professions Commission. (1998). *Recreating health professional practice for new professionals for the 21st century.* Washington, DC: Pew Health Professions Commission.

Spreitzer, G., & Porath, C. (2012, January–February). Creating sustainable performance. *Harvard Business Review, 90*(1–2), 92–99.

Whitney, D., Trosten-Bloom, A., & Radu, K. (2010). *Appreciative leadership: Focus on what works to drive winning performance.* New York, NY: McGraw Hill.

World Health Organization (WHO). (2006). *The world health report 2006: Working together for health.* Geneva, Switzerland: The World Health Organization.

Zolno, S. (2007). Towards a healthy world: Meeting the challenges of the 21st century. *Linkage,* (34), 14.

Zolno, S., & Skillman, R. (2011). *Coaching certification in whole system IQ and appreciative inquiry.* Vaushon, WA: The Leading Clinic.

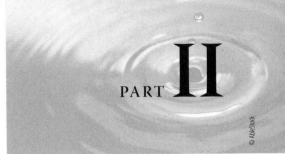

PART **II**

© AbleStock

Relationship-Centered Leadership Activities

Activity 1: Myers-Briggs—Your Leadership Behavior Under Stress and at Your Best

Using the following tables, write a profile regarding your leadership behaviors at your best and under stress. Think about a recent incident in a group where you were "at your best" and you were "under stress." How did you feel? How did the other group members respond? How can you use these insights to further develop your leadership skills?

ISTJ, ISFJ		ESTP, ESFP	
Dominant, Introverted Sensing		Dominant, Extroverted Sensing	
At one's best	Under stress	At one's best	Under stress
• Are selective, choose the right facts • Have excellent recall • Are sure and certain • Reflect before acting • Communicate perspective to others	• Fixate on the right facts • Obsess with minute data • Are dogmatic • Become paralyzed—take no action • Shut down	• See and think; then do or say • Are active • Are talkative, sociable • Are straightforward and clear • Pay attention to detail	• Speak and act without thinking • Are hyperactive • Chatter and disturb others • Are blunt and curt • Are pedantic

INTJ, INFJ		ENTP, ENFP	
Dominant, Introverted Intuition		**Dominant, Extroverted Intuition**	
At one's best	**Under stress**	**At one's best**	**Under stress**
• Are problem solvers • Are visionary • See connections • Make patterns • Have in-depth theory	• Are arrogant, do not admit dependence on others • Have visions detached from reality • Are overly complex, everything is connected • Force data to fit • Will not ask for help	• Form global pictures • Are innovative • Are enthusiastic • See possibilities • Are flexible • Are fast paced	• Are obsessed with links between things • Are different just for the sake of novelty • Are frantic • Dither—cannot decide between too many options • Spin out of control

ISTP, INTP		ESTJ, ENTJ	
Dominant, Introverted Thinking		**Dominant, Extroverted Thinking**	
At one's best	**Under stress**	**At one's best**	**Under stress**
• Persistently search for the truth • Have depth of concentration • Are logical • Are objective • Are self-motivated	• Obsessively search for the truth • Are lost in concentration • Only his or her logic accepted • Become totally detached • Are driven—like a machine out of control	• Are cool headed • Are rational • Possesses clarity • Are logical • Are analytical	• Are cold, detached • Think everything must be rational • Oversimplify for the sake of clarity • Insist upon logic • Dominate others by criticizing them

ISFP, INFP		ESFJ, ENFJ	
Dominant, Introverted Feeling		**Dominant, Extroverted Feeling**	
At one's best	**Under stress**	**At one's best**	**Under stress**
• Are empathetic • Think people matter, including themselves • Are independent • Are sensitive • Are idealistic	• Are rescuers • Carry the weight of the world on their shoulders • Isolate selves • Are hypersensitive • Are demagogic—thinking their ideals are the only ones	• Are encouraging • Are interested in others • Seek harmony • Are outward looking • Are people and relationship oriented	• Are insistent; e.g., "you will enjoy this" • Are intrusive • Ignore problems for surface harmony • Have a lack of focus • Are overburdened, overidentified with others

Data from: Hirsh, S. (1996). *Work It Out: Clues for Solving People Problems at Work.* Boston: Nicholas Brealey Publishing.

Activity 2: Best Manager

Take a moment to think about the best and worst managers you have ever had throughout your working life. What adjectives would you use to describe your worst manager?

- Describe the specific behaviors this person demonstrated.
- What effect did this person have on you and others?

What adjectives would you use to describe your best manager?

- Describe the specific behaviors this person demonstrated.
- What effect did this person have on you and others?

Think about yourself as a leader. What three adjectives would you use to describe yourself as a leader?

- Describe your behavior when you are leading.
- How do you look and feel when you are leading?

Activity 3: Leadership Learning Journey

The leadership learning journey is a series of activities. Complete them in sequence. Begin with your lifeline and continue until you have a completed leadership learning plan. The leadership learning journey steps are lifeline, values sort, circle of life, back from the future, and the leadership learning plan.

Lifeline Exercise

Effective leaders reflect on all aspects of their lives. Reflective analysis of life experiences can assist in goal setting and charting a course for personal and professional development.

PURPOSE: To take a reflective journey to the past to explore in-depth impact, emotionally engaging experiences and the lessons learned from those experiences.

Instructions

1. On a blank sheet of paper, draw a horizontal line.
2. On the left, write the year you were born. On the right, note today's date and finish the line with an arrow pointing to the future.
3. Along your lifeline, make a note of:
   - Important events in your life
   - Transition points
   - High moments
   - Low moments
   - Things you are proud of
   - Things you are sorry about
4. Include both personal and professional events and issues.

Be sure to pay attention to the emotions you feel as you fill in your lifeline. A sample lifeline is shown in **Figure PII-1**.

Values Sort

Values are the foundation of who we are, what we do, how we feel about ourselves, our family and friends, our work or career, and how we interact with others. They affect our beliefs about what is right or wrong, and we often make decisions based on our values.

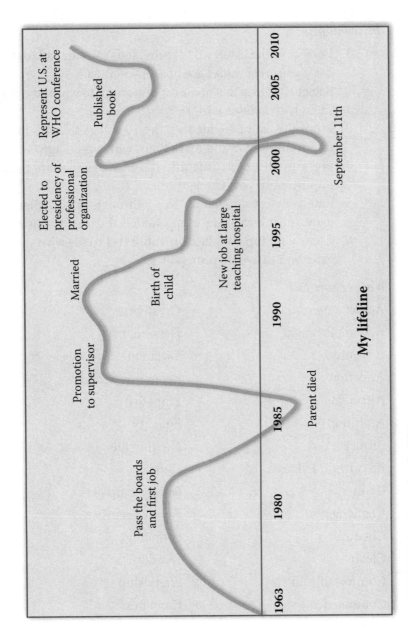

FIGURE PII-1   Example of a lifeline.

Instructions:

1. Look over the list of values provided. You can add to this list if your real values are not represented.
2. Select 15 values that are most important to you and mark them with an asterisk (*).
3. From the list of 15, identify the 10 values that are most important to you and mark them with a plus sign (+).
4. From the list of 10, identify the 5 values that are most important to you. Circle those 5.
5. Rate your list of 5 values No. 1 through No. 5, where 1 is the most important value and 5 is the least important.
6. Circle your top 10 values on **Table II-1** to see what motivates you to live by your values.

Values Sort List

Achievement	Creativity
Accomplishment	Dependability
Adventure	Discipline
Affection	Economic Security
Altruism	Empathy
Ambition	Equality
Beauty	Exciting life
Broad-mindedness	Fame
Calm	Family happiness
Challenging	Family security
Cheerful	Forgiving
Clean	Freedom
Comfortable life	Friendship
Competence	Happiness
Competitiveness	Health
Contribution	Helpfulness
Cooperation	Inner harmony
Courage	Innovation

Integrity

Intellectual

Involvement

Logic

Loving

Loyalty

Mature love

National security

Order

Peace (no conflict)

Personal development

Pleasure

Politeness

Power

Recognition

Religion

Respect for life

Responsibility

Restraint

Risk taking

Salvation

Self-control

Self-respect

Serenity

Spirituality

Stability

Status

Success

Wealth

Wisdom

_____

_____

_____

Rank the five values most important to you (1 = most important, etc.).

1. _____

2. _____

3. _____

4. _____

5. _____

What is Motivating My Values?

Motivation is what incentivizes you toward action. When you are lying in bed in the morning, what inspires you to get up . . . getting something done (accomplishment), seeing your children (relationships), etc.? Your values are often a product of your core motivation. Circle your top 10 values in Table II-1 to help you identify what motivates you.

TABLE II-1   Value Motivation

Motivation	Values		
Relationships	Adventure	Equality	Loyalty
	Affection	Family happiness	Mature love
	Altruism	Forgiving	Peace (no conflict)
	Broad mindedness	Friendship	Politeness
	Cooperation	Helpfulness	Respect for life
	Dependability	Involvement	
	Empathy	Loving	
Accomplishment	Achievement	Competence	Personal development
	Accomplishment	Competitiveness	Recognition
	Ambition	Economic security	Risk taking
	Adventure	Fame	Status
	Challenge	Innovation	Success
Influence	Contribution	Family security	Restraint
	Courage	Freedom	Stability
	Discipline	National security	Wealth
	Order	Responsibility	
Well-being, self-expression and style	Beauty	Health	Salvation
	Calm	Inner harmony	Self-control
	Cheerful	Integrity	Self-respect
	Clean	Intellectual	Serenity
	Comfortable life	Logic	Spirituality
	Creativity	Pleasure	Wisdom
	Exciting life	Power	
	Happiness	Religion	

Data from: Simon, S., Howe, L., and Kirschenbaum, H. (1995) *Values Clarification.* New York, NY: Grand Central Publishing; and McClelland, D. (1988). *Human Motivation.* New York, NY: Cambridge University Press.

Does this line up with your motivations? What else motivates you?

Circles of Life

PURPOSE: To identify current state and future priorities.

We all have multiple competing priorities in our lives. Sometimes it is helpful to take stock of where we are spending our time and compare this to how we ideally would like to spend our time. For this exercise, list the categories of activities that are important to you. The list may look like this:

- Exercise
- Work
- Spending time with my family
- Learning and education
- Spiritual practice
- Entertainment (e.g., movies, TV, social networking)

Now draw circles that represent the amount of time you spend in each area. Some will naturally intersect as shown in the following example:

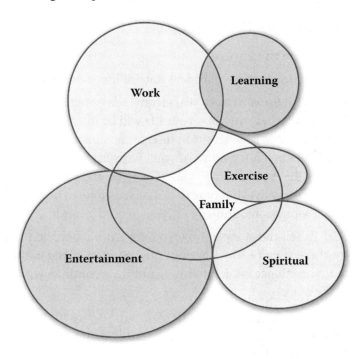

If you like, fill in the percentages of the time you spend in these categories in the following table. Add and delete categories for your Ideal column but be realistic (i.e., you probably do need to spend a good percentage of your time at work, but you may want to have your work overlap more with learning).

Category	% of Time You Spend Now	Ideal Percentage of Time

Now draw your ideal circles of life.

Back from the Future

PURPOSE: Identify your ideal state of life 5–10 years from now.

Part 1: Fast forward to 10 years from today. Spend a few moments imagining what you hope your life will be like. Focus specifically on your role as a leader on an interprofessional team. Write a few words or sketch a picture of what your life will be like. You can include the type of person you hope to be, the people around you, the place you live, the type of leader you hope to be, your professional aspirations, and any other aspects of your life.

Part 2: Tell the story of how you got from where you are today to where you are 10 years from now. Start by filling in the blanks in first sentence, which follows, and then continue with the rest of the story.

Today is _____ (today's date, month, and this year +10).
I am now _____ (describe yourself 10 years from today). This is how I got here:

Leadership Learning Plan

PURPOSE: To articulate vision, learning goals, milestones, and action steps.

Learning goals should be challenging and should include building on your strengths, as well as overcoming limitations as you develop these goals. Specific, measureable, actionable, realistic, and time-bounded (SMART) goals are:

- *Specific:* A specific goal is better than a general one. Learning a new language is general. Learning Chinese is specific. Being a better leader is general; listening to team member input and feedback is more specific.
- *Measurable:* How will you measure your accomplishment? What will success look like? Examples include: I will complete the first three chapters of Chinese in *Rosetta Stone* in the next 6 months; and I will articulate three messages (input/ feedback) that I have heard from my colleagues each month.
- *Actionable:* Can you take action on this goal? Do you have the ability and resources you need to learn a new language? Are you approaching patient care from a client-centered and interdisciplinary way and do team members give you input and feedback?
- *Realistic:* Are you willing and able to achieve this goal? Do you really have time to learn Chinese? Do you spend time with

Leadership competency I need to develop: Continuously work to be a more strategic leader	
Action steps:	**Timeline:**
1. Read "Good to Great"	1. Finish by December 2012
2. Take a course in how to give feedback	2. January 2013
3. Create a coach who can help me: my boss; my colleague; my friend; my relative	3. By January 2013

FIGURE PII-2   Sample of a Leadership Learning Goal.

team members, and are you creating a safe environment for this type of communication?

■ *Time bounded:* What is your time frame for completing this? Examples might be: In one year, I will be able to hold a simple conversation in Chinese; and in three months I will know enough about what members of my interdisciplinary team think to respond to the input with actions.

My Goals:

1. _____
2. _____
3. _____
4. _____

My New Leadership Learning Plan

Leadership Competency I Need to Develop (Goal No. 1):	
Action steps:	*Timeline:*
1.	1.
2.	2.
3.	3.

Leadership Competency I Need to Develop (Goal No. 2):	
Action steps:	*Timeline:*
1.	1.
2.	2.
3.	3.

Leadership Competency I Need to Develop (Goal No. 3):	
Action steps:	*Timeline:*
1.	1.
2.	2.
3.	3.

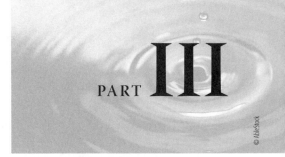

Building and Sustaining Collaborative Interprofessional Teams

"We prepare for an unknown future by creating strong and sustainable relationships . . . and by building resilient communities . . . human beings are caring, generous and want to be together. We have learned that whatever the problem, community is the answer."

Margaret J. Wheatley, the Berkana Institute

Chapter 7: Leveraging Diversity

Chapter 8: Facilitating a Collaborative Culture

Chapter 9: Generative Practices

Part III Activities

Leveraging Diversity

Learning Objectives

1. Differentiate surface-level and deep-level diversity.
2. Apply communication strategies, such as deep listening, that recognize and respect the diversity of interprofessional healthcare teams.
3. Explain how negative capability fosters innovative thought and creative problem solving in diverse groups.
4. Manage conflict.
5. Create a psychologically safe team environment.

Teams reflect the thriving diversity of our communities. The amount and outward appearance of diversity varies organizationally, regionally, and internationally, and understanding its impact on teamwork is vital for any team leader or member (Knippenberg & Schippers, 2007). Mannix and Neale (2005) suggest the following six broad diversity categories: social identity, knowledge and skills, values and beliefs, personality, organizational and community, and social network (**Table 7-1**).

All of these aspects of diversity are salient to interdisciplinary healthcare teams and have been classified by some at the surface

TABLE 7-1 Mannix and Neale Diversity Categories

Category	Examples
Social identity	Gender, ethnicity, religious identity, sexual orientation
Knowledge and skills	Educational background, functional knowledge
Values and beliefs	Cultural background—family of origin, generation, personal history of experiences
Personality	Cognitive styles, temperament
Organizational and community	Status-like placement in organizational hierarchy, tenure, social-economic, respect for profession in society
Social network	Friends and work-related network of associates, family members

Data from: Mannix, E. & Neale, M.A. (2005). What makes a difference? The promise and reality of diverse teams in organizations. *Psychological Science in the Public Interest,* 6, 31–55.

(demographic) level or deep (psychological) level (Harrison, et al, 2002). Others define diversity to include any dimension of social identity where there is a history of intergroup prejudice, discrimination, or oppression (race, ethnicity, gender, religion, sexual orientation, nationality) (Ely & Roberts, 2008). The observable differences (surface) and variations in subjective perceptions

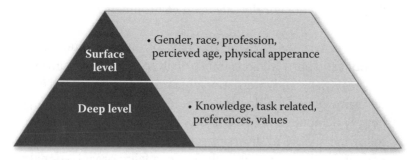

FIGURE 7-1 Dimensions of diversity: surface and deep level.

Data from: Mannix, E. & Neale, M.A. (2005) "What makes a difference? The promise and reality of diverse teams in organizations." Psychological Science in the Public Interest, 6:31-55.

(psychological) are the sources of many challenges and opportunities in interdisciplinary healthcare teams.

Surface-Level Diversity

Surface-level diversity or demographic diversity can be defined as attributes that are physical, not easily changeable, and almost immediately observable. Age, race/ethnicity, and gender are all considered surface diversity. Social categories like organizational function, professional background, and organizational status are also considered surface diversity. Most importantly, it is well established that these characteristics often form the basis for stereotypes—social classifications involving prescribed patterns of thought attitudes and behaviors (Fiske, 2000). Surface-level diversity has been shown to negatively impact team function resulting in social isolation, diminished communication, lack of attachment, reduced cohesion, and poor performance. Fortunately, it has also been shown that as teams work together longer, the increased opportunities for interaction around common goals tends to mitigate the negative effects of surface diversity (Harrison et al., 2002).

Deep-Level Diversity

Deep-level diversity or psychological diversity is defined as personality, value, and attitude differences among team members. These are not immediately apparent but impact team function (Harrison et al., 2002). Professional training and strength of professional identity often reinforce the personality, values, and attitudes that influence an individual's choice of profession. All of these factors impact professional behavior. For example, a physician's primary interest is the health and well-being of the individual patient, while an administrator's responsibility is the viability of the hospital system. Both are legitimate and necessary orientations that may occasionally be sources of conflict. Not surprisingly, individuals prefer to interact with those who share similar psychological characteristics because that interaction validates their commonly held beliefs, affect, and expressed behaviors (Swann, Stein-Seroussi, & Geisler, 1992).

Integrating the Levels of Diversity

Interestingly, while teams that are homogeneous at the surface and deep levels perform better in the early stages of a team's work life, more diverse teams—given the time to gain more information about each other and to work on group processes—are better at identifying problems and generating solutions. Ely and Roberts (2008) suggest that focusing on team goals such as improving patient care, creating better continuing education structures, or implementing new technology is an effective strategy for channeling diverse perspectives.

Each individual has a personal worldview based on myriad social, psychological, and economic factors, and additional biases are imposed by professional or disciplinary culture. The lenses through which each member of a healthcare team views interdisciplinary teamwork may vary widely. For instance, every member of the team may have a differing view of who is considered part of the team. Is it the physician and the nurse? The physician, the nurse, and the therapy staff? What about the pharmacist and the health information manager? The dietician? Are the clerical staff included? Transportation? In addition, a physician may view the team as governed by hierarchy. Members who are viewed as having lesser status may be valued more for their ability to carry out the directives of those who have more status than they are for their ability to provide innovative or additional insight into patient care. Occupational therapists and physical therapists may see the roles between team members as more flexible and be more comfortable collaborating and negotiating disciplinary boundaries. Some mental health professionals may view themselves as autonomous and only engage other professionals as needed. What and how information is communicated is governed by each team member's perception of the team's composition, purpose, roles, and responsibilities.

The more closely aligned the members' perceptions, the higher the probability of optimum team performance and outcomes. At the heart of highly functional healthcare teams lies mutual respect born out of an interest in continually learning about each other, committment to team goals and making optimum functioning the norm. Reflection becomes the impetus and result of learning. Open communication, reflection, respect, and continuous learning facilitate the accumulation of social capital that sustains high-performance teams and organizations (Ghaye, 2005).

The need for a complex array of services such as medical, therapeutic, pharmaceutical, nutritional, social, and pastoral services and clerical, data management, transportation, infection control, medical supplies, and equipment management highlights the interdependence of all the stakeholders in the healthcare arena. For example, productivity in the occupational and physical therapy departments might be highly dependent on the efficiency of transportation services. Leaders and members who employ inclusionary practices such as soliciting input from all stakeholders in the healthcare process, recognizing successful practices and consistently facilitating positive communication create psychological safety, which encourages participation and engagement in collaborative healthcare practices. Mindful attention to relationship building mitigates the tensions that accompany interdependence. In the following case study, the physician was cognizant that her view of the patient might be incomplete and the transporter felt that his opinion was valuable and relevant to the successful patient outcome. As a result, the patient received safe and effective care.

High staff turnover presents a challenge for those who would attempt to develop strong healthcare teams. The culture of positive regard that is modeled by the leader and senior team members and adopted by all the members of the team creates a trusting and respectful work environment that transcends the behavior of particular individuals and facilitates the honest reflection and inquiry that is the bedrock of quality improvement in health care. By institutionalizing feedback strategies, power sharing becomes the responsibility of leaders as well as members who provide each other with constructive opinions and supportive advice. Meetings that are structured to facilitate universal contribution will demonstrate institutional valuation of collaboration. Senior

---

CASE STUDY

A physician was preparing the discharge orders for a patient who would need help with dressing and transferring from bed to wheelchair. It was expected that she would be discharged to the care of her daughter. At the weekly meeting, the physician polled the members of the team asking that each person share any information they had about the patient. A member of the transportation staff assigned to the rehabilitation unit had reported to the nurse that when he was transporting the patient to her final therapy session, she shared that her daughter had been injured in a car accident the previous day and she was in a neck brace. Further investigation by social services corroborated the report and orders to discharge the patient to a skilled nursing facility were issued.

---

team members who hold high-status positions and/or as those who have been on the job longest have a unique opportunity to enculturate new team members by modeling relationship-building behaviors that facilitate interpersonal trust, respect, and active engagement in collaborator team efforts. A psychologically safe work environment is an important factor in staff retention and mitigates the risk associated with behaviors that bridge status differentials such as suggesting new procedures, offering unsolicited feedback, or sharing innovative ideas. The return on this investment in social capital is an engaged, loyal, stable workforce and a vibrant, innovative work environment. As the tenure of team members within a position increases, so does their communication and tendency to pay less attention to status differentials. As status barriers fade and team-wide collaboration increases, opportunities for creative problem solving and innovation abound. The benefits of an experienced, competent, loyal, engaged, and stable workforce cannot be underestimated in any circumstances. In health care, the well-being of patients depends on it (IOM, 2001, 2002, 2003). Time spent training leaders and members of interprofessional healthcare teams to be inclusive and to foster psychological safety is time well spent and should be incorporated into staff development initiatives for new and experienced staff (Nembhard & Edmondson, 2006).

The highly specialized training that is the hallmark of traditional health professional education places a premium on knowing and leaves little room for understanding the perspectives of multiple disciplines. Those professionals who have a negative capability or an ability to not know are more comfortable working in the ambiguous space between disciplines and more likely to encourage innovative thought and creative solutions to complex problems (Hammick et al., 2009; Whitney, et al., 2010). Leaders who attain a comfort level with the tension inherent in not knowing encourage all the members of their teams to question the status quo, think creatively, and seek new ways to approach problem solving (French, Simpson, & Harvey, 2001).

Knowing when to defer to the expertise of others is a valuable trait for leaders/members of interdisciplinary healthcare teams. The strength of the team lies in its ability to leverage the skills of multiple disciplines toward the common goal of client-centered care. While individual members of the interdisciplinary team have a comfort level with traditionally prescribed roles and responsibilities, they must be cognizant of the limits of their knowledge and capabilities and reach beyond disciplinary boundaries in order to facilitate relationships and client-centered versus disciplinary-centered practice.

By deep listening—refocusing our attention on the orientation of others—instead of talking and by asking questions rather than making statements, leaders/members of healthcare teams can transform disciplinary boundaries from spaces of conflict to spaces of new learning and innovation in relationship-based, patient-centered care (French, Simpson, & Harvey, 2001; Gray, 2008; Klein, 2010). It appears that the most effective leaders are those whose allegiance to group goals supersedes personal goals or who have a strong other orientation. Gray (2008) suggests that leadership behaviors in well-functioning interdisciplinary groups can be demonstrated through cognitive, structural, and procedural tasks. Cognitive tasks often take the form of appreciative forms of inquiry where the focus is placed on how the team can make best practice the norm rather than how the team can avoid mistakes. With specialized training comes greater natural resistance to alternative methods and approaches as well as

REFLECTION: *A Different View*

- Choose an event (work meeting, speech, event from the evening news).
- Ask your colleagues to describe their interpretation of the event.
- How many different explanations did you hear?
- What did you hear that surprised you?
- How did it change your perspective?

greater difficulty communicating approaches to others who are not similarly trained. Bridging the gaps between the disciplines is often a key role that healthcare leaders play for their organization (Garman, 2010). Establishing strong social networks within the team and with stakeholders outside of the team are structural or bridge-building behaviors that serve to neutralize power and disciplinary differentials and garner universal engagement of all team members. Procedural tasks such as the design of meetings, the establishment of standards for information exchange, and conflict management ensure constructive and productive decision making, innovative problem solving, and conflict resolution among team members.

REFLECTION: *Listening with New Eyes*

- Think of someone with whom you often disagree.
- Think of a topic in which both of you are interested.
- Ask him/her for an opinion/explanation on that topic. Sit quietly and listen to the answer without saying anything for a while.
- How might you encourage the person to just keep telling you about his/her perspective?
- What are the actual differences in your perspectives? What are the similarities?
- What surprised you?

Managing Conflict

Health professionals often find themselves in positions that require negotiations with their peers, their superiors, and their subordinates. The discussions frequently focus on varied views regarding what constitutes best practice. Studer (2003) points out that proactive leaders negotiate with their constituencies in order to establish a set of agreed-upon objective criteria that represents a commonly held view of excellence. In the healthcare arena, objective measurements—whether they are patient satisfaction surveys, achievement of stated goals within a specific time frame, or a decrease in cost or increase in referrals—can serve

---

CASE STORY: *Identifying Outcome Options*

Many special needs pre-school children had been referred to private programs for intensive early intervention which included physical therapy, occupational therapy and speech therapy. When they reached school age, they received therapy services within their school systems. Parents who were accustomed to individual daily therapy sessions in the private settings lobbied for similar services within the school system. Teachers were concerned about the disruption that pulling children out for the various therapies might cause. The school based therapists were doubtful that they could effectively manage such a large case load. Administrators had to deal with the restrictions of limited space, time and financial resources.

All sides had the opportunity to share their legitimate, but sometimes opposing, concerns. During the discussions, everyone was asked to express their main concern. Not surprisingly, they shared a genuine desire to provide efficient and effective services for the children.

The commonly held desire for efficient and effective services was the point of departure for productive discussions about alternative, less direct approaches to therapy that were more suited to the regular school schedule such as program and case consultation, monitoring, technical assistance and in-service programming for teachers and hands-on workshops for parents.

In the long term, many of the tools and techniques that were shared could be incorporated into daily home and school life—making both environments inherently therapeutic and very effective in facilitating the childrens' development.

as manifestations of best practice in action or excellent performance. Once objective criteria are in place, the team can focus on the key behaviors that contribute to excellent performance.

Fisher and Ury (1991) expand upon Studer's notion by noting that commonly agreed upon objective criteria can help inform the development of a number of alternative solutions that are consistent with the interests of the other side. This demonstration of a willingness to be persuaded—of being open to new ideas— can engender similar attitudes in those whom you wish to persuade. A good negotiator assumes the role of problem solver rather than adversary and is patient, flexible and creative in the search for mutually beneficial solutions that are based on principles rather than positions. There is no doubt that this deliberate, strategic method of interaction requires time and skills such as patience, self regulation, empathy, listening, communicating, objectivity and logic.

Questions tend to generate answers while statements tend to generate resistance so the successful negotiator should concentrate on asking good questions rather than making statements (Fisher & Ury, 1991). The more skillful one becomes in asking people for feedback and advice, the more successful one becomes

---

REFLECTION: *Workplace Negotiation*

Every day, we all engage in negotiations—big and small—in our workplace. Think of an issue that you and a colleague or colleagues disagree about. Take on the role of problem solver rather than adversary.

- What is the issue that has to be negotiated?
- What are some of the interests that influence the positions of the people involved in the negotiation?
- What are some of the objective criteria that might be used to help guide the negotiation?
- List all of the outcome options for the above issues/problems that are possible in your setting.
- How would you and your colleagues feel about the possible outcomes of this negotiation?

in gathering the data that is most important to them. Focusing on another's felt need (not on personalities or emotions) helps to facilitate successful outcomes that contribute to excellent service delivery.

More often than not, successful patient outcomes depend on health professionals' ability to adjust their view to accommodate the views of others and negotiate many disciplinary perspectives . . . all of which are legitimate and meaningful to the progress of the patient.

Institutional excellence and effective leadership of interdisciplinary teams depends on the integration of various points of view. Communication tools such as team meetings, performance evaluations, productivity logs, and surveys are valuable means by which team members can share their perspectives and increase their effectiveness. It is within these day-to-day interactions that interprofessional curiosity, active listening, and principled negotiation techniques will afford the opportunity to engage in the ongoing process of establishing the most important things to the team. The consistent and reliable measurement of outcomes related to the important things will help all constituencies constantly assess their progress on the journey to excellence and provide clarification regarding if and when the definition of *the important things* needs to be reassessed. So, for example, a team may agree that it is important for soon-to-be discharged diabetic patients to receive training regarding wound care, but the administrator is concerned about financial and space restrictions, transportation services are concerned about getting patients to yet another location, and nurses and therapists have concerns about integrating specific techniques into the client's daily schedule.

REFLECTION: *What is Most Important to the Team?*

- How can you establish what is important from your institution's, supervisor's, or other team member's point of view? How will you go beyond your *assumptions* of what they think?

- How will this alter your perception of what the important things are?

CASE STORY: *Interdisciplinary Teams, Building Bridges, and Culture Change in Southern Africa*

We worked with interdisciplinary teams who were involved in addressing various aspects of the HIV/AIDS crisis in southern Africa. These teams were made up of 100 individuals who were doctors, nurses, traditional healers, social workers, educators, United Nations relief workers, government officials, and media specialists communication professionals. Less than a decade before this meeting, many of these same people lived under apartheid, where roles and functions were strictly prescribed and biases ran deep. This diverse group of people needed to work together to reduce the spread of HIV/AIDS, deliver care to persons already infected with the disease, and distribute medicine over a vast geographic area where 30–40% of the population was affected by the epidemic.

The ultimate goal of this work was to shift the culture surrounding HIV/AIDS from stigma to respect and caring, from despair to hope, and from secrecy to self-disclosure. Workshops were designed to train the 100 team members as well as facilitators who could take the workshop design to others. Using experiential learning methods and appreciative inquiry techniques, participants conducted their own needs assessments and participated in focused sessions on emotional intelligence, gender and age differences. They explored leadership, team dynamics, and the causes and effects of stigma and how to foster behavior change.

Through small- and large-group activities, people built trust and revealed personal life stories. Barriers between heritage, histories, and professions were crossed, and people found that they bonded across roles. Bonding as human beings went beyond the surface of teacher, doctor, nurse, social worker, and public policy maker. The establishment of collective goals and hope for the future transcended the pain of history. An appreciation for individual talents and the power of the collective evolved.

The collective energy that was unleashed by this experience spilled out into the community. Participants implemented their learning through projects such as a media campaign to encourage the use of antiretroviral drugs (ARVs) undertaken by a young organizer of an AIDS support group, nurses, educators, and journalists. A compilation of videotaped interviews of southern Africans expressing their opinions of what they thought would help to rid the stigma of HIV/AIDS was created by a TV journalist, fund raiser, police officer, and social worker with funds secured from the Coca-Cola Company.

Every participant emerged from the training experience as a changed person—a change agent who continues to change the culture by transforming the lives and perspectives of others.

—Felice Tilin, President of GroupWorks Consulting and Delores Mason, President of 2YourWellBeing

GUIDELINES *for Managing Diversity in Interdisciplinary Teams*

Moderate power dynamics:
- Make sure everyone has a voice.
- Start meetings with check-ins from all members.
- Rotate responsibility for leading meetings.

Focus on common professional values and goals:
- Create a common team identity. Take time to establish and articulate who the team is and what it stands for. Establish what is important to the team.
- Share variations in perspectives regarding commonly held values and goals.

Decide how decisions will be made:
- Decision making depends on the task. Some tasks will require the expert to make the final decision. Some tasks may require consensus. Some will require a majority vote.

Create a safe, transparent environment:
- Establish ground rules for meetings and interactions and stick to them.
- Spend time getting to know each other beyond professional roles.

Recognize the value of well-managed conflict:
- Seek the principle behind the position. Ask questions such as, "how did you arrive at that conclusion?"
- Do not defend your position. Ask for feedback. Making statements tends to generate resistance while asking questions tends to generate answers.

Recognize and reward success.
- Set up a time to articulate celebrate team successes.

The common valuation of patient education serves as the point of departure for a discussion of all the possibilities, and the team agrees that a series of electronic training manuals, FAQ sites, or electronic discussion environments where questions, answers, and suggestions can be shared in an asynchronous manner might address all concerns as well as the most important thing in this case—patient education.

References

Ely, R. J., & Roberts, L. M. (2008). Shifting frames in team-diversity research: From difference to relationships. In AP Brief, *Diversity at Work* (pp. 175–201). New York, NY: Cambridge University Press.

Fisher, R., & Ury, W. (1991). *Getting to yes: Negotiating agreement without giving in* (2nd ed.). New York, NY: Penguin Books.

Fiske, S. T. (2000). Interdependence and reduction of prejudice. In S. Oskamp (Ed.), *Reducing prejudice and discrimination* (pp. 115–135). Mahwah, NJ: Erlbaum.

French, Simpson, & Harvey, (June 2001,). *Negative capability: The key to creative leadership.* Presented at the International Society for the Psychoanalytic Study of Organizations symposia. Paris, France.

Garman, A. (2010). Leadership development in the interdisciplinary context. In B. Freshman, L. Rubino, & Y. Chassiakos (Eds.), *Collaboration across the disciplines in health care.* Sudbury, MA: Jones and Bartlett Learning.

Ghaye, T. (2005). *Developing the reflective healthcare team.* Oxford, UK: Blackwell Publishing, Ltd.

Gray, B. (2008). Enhancing transdisciplinary research through collaborative leadership. *American Journal of Preventive Medicine, 35*(2S), s124–s132.

Hammick, M., Freeth, D., Copperman, J., & Goodsman, D. (2009). *Being interprofessional.* Malden, MA: Polity Press.

Harrison, D., Price, K., Gavin, J., & Florey, K. (2002). Group functioning. *Academy of Management Journal, 45*(5), 1029–1045.

Institutes of Medicine. (2001). *Crossing the quality chasm: A new health system for the 21st Century.* Washington, DC: National Academy Press.

Institutes of Medicine. (2002). *Who will keep the public healthy? Educating public health.* Washington, DC: National Academy Press.

Institutes of Medicine. (2003). *Health professions education: A bridge to quality.* Washington, DC: National Academy Press.

Klein, J. (2010). *Creating interdisciplinary campus cultures: A model for strength and sustainability.* San Francisco, CA: Jossey-Bass.

Knippenberg, D., & Schippers, M. (2007). Work group diversity. *Annual Review of Psychology, 58,* 515–541.

Mannix, E., & Neale, M. A. (2005). What makes a difference? The promise and reality of diverse teams in organizations. *Psychological Science in the Public Interest, 6,* 31–55.

Milliken, F., & Martins, L. (1996). Searching for common threads: Understanding the multiple effects of diversity in organizational groups. *Academy of Management Review, 21*(2), 402–433.

Nembhard, I., & Edmondson, A. (2006). Making it safe: The effects of leader inclusiveness and professional status on psychological safety and improvement efforts in health care teams. *Journal of Organizational Behavior, 27,* 941–966.

Studer, Q. (2003). *Hardwiring excellence: Purpose, worthwhile work, making a difference.* Gulf Breeze, FL: Fire Starter Publishing.

Swann, W., Stein-Seroussi, A., & Giesler, B. (1992). Why people self-verify. *Journal of Personality and Social Psychology, 62,* 392–401.

Whitney, D., Trosten-Bloom, A., & Radu, K. (2010). *Appreciative leadership: Focus on what works to drive winning performance.* New York, NY: McGraw-Hill.

CHAPTER 8

Facilitating a Collaborative Culture

Learning Objectives

1. Analyze collaborative leadership behaviors in real-life situations.
2. Analyze team cultures.
3. Employ positive communication and productive, interprofessional dialogue to facilitate team function.
4. Identify boundary-spanning activities that support collaborative cultures.
5. Understand the dynamics of successful interprofessional healthcare teams.

Every organization has its own unique spoken and unspoken rules that define the culture. Culture is often simply stated as, "the way we work around here." Cultures are formed and change through a variety of environmental events, leadership, and experiences. Dramatic and sometimes traumatic events impact the way cultures operate much the same way that the environment impacts personality in individuals. The way leaders respond to these events also shapes the culture. Edgar Schein (1986) defined culture using the following three levels:

1. *Artifacts:* These are the things you can easily see on the surface. How people behave is an artifact of culture.
2. *Espoused values:* These are the stated goals, philosophies, and values of an organization or group. Vision, mission, and values statements published on webpages, on posters, or in team charters are examples of espoused values.
3. *Basic assumptions and values:* These are the unconscious workings that underlie the core behaviors of a group. Shifting from a primarily hierarchical, disciplinary-centered culture to a more relationship- and patient-centered, collaborative culture is one of the primary challenges for healthcare systems.

Team cultures that value and actively seek each member's contribution can only inspire collaboration, commitment, and active engagement in the achievement of common goals (Wheatley, 2005, 2006; Whitney, Trosten-Bloom, & Radu, 2010). Successful team leadership is, at its heart, an affirmation of the need for human beings to contribute and collaborate in a positive manner. Zolno (2007) perceives leadership as a generative act that is facilitated by a personal sense of self-worth, hope, and capability. Individuals who develop their own sense of worth, hopes, and capabilities can, through positive communication, transmit those values to others. Affirmative cultures are created and sustained through positive, rather than negative, dialogues and groups who demonstrate a higher ratio of positive language tend to be more open to new ideas, more creative, and productive. As feelings

REFLECTION: *Cultural Cues*

- What are some of the artifacts of your organization/team?
- What are the espoused values of your organization/team?
- If a friend was joining your organization/team and he wanted to know how to succeed, what would you tell him about the unspoken values and assumptions of your organization/team?

of self-efficacy emerge and grow, so does the perceived range of choices and possibility for action (Frederickson, 2003, 2009).

Like a pebble dropped into a pond, acts of affirmative leadership begin with the self and radiate out to impact other individuals, groups, organizations, and local and global communities. The result is the distribution of leadership behaviors beyond the designated leader and a facilitation of a culture of possibilities—a collective willingness to try new things and a more equal sharing of responsibility for goals and outcomes. Not surprisingly, this concept is associated not only with best practices in interdisciplinary healthcare teams but also in a wide range of highly profitable business endeavors (Anchor, 2012; Briskin et al, 2009; Fox, 2012; IOM, 2001, 2002, 2003; Pew, 1998; Spietzer & Porath, 2012).

Creating and maintaining a collaborative culture is an important aspect of a professional orientation—no matter what the discipline or position in the organization. The mindfulness, hope, and compassion that are the hallmarks of effective leaders are also instrumental in facilitating collaborative cultures. Members of the healthcare professions are well schooled in the aspects of mindfulness, hope, and compassion—as they apply to their relationship with their patients. Compassion and empathy for others are often the motivation for pursuing a healthcare career. Good clinical reasoning requires focused examination of objective clinical information in combination with mindful, in-the-moment analysis of the unique, subjective illness experience of each patient. Hope—the firm belief in the capability of the health professions and the resilience of the human spirit to overcome adversity and positively affect the quality of patient's lives—lies at the very core of every health profession. The challenge for leaders and members of healthcare teams is to understand that it is their responsibility to take a leadership stance and employ these qualities in the interactions with coworkers, superiors, and subordinates as well as with their patients.

Members of high performing teams perceive their work environment as having high levels of flexibility, responsibility, standards, rewards, clarity, and team commitment. They feel that new ideas are welcomed, their expertise is trusted, accountability and excellence are the norm, expectations are clear, and there is a commonality of purpose (Spreier, Fontaine, & Malloy, 2006). The designated leader of the team sets the tone by modeling collaborative behaviors but also actively coaches team members by learning to listen, learning to ask powerful questions, and creating a safe environment based on trust and confidentiality.

Leaders facilitate the team's capacity to adapt by encouraging diverse perspectives. Members who take a leadership stance do so by practicing a professional assertiveness that allows them to offer their unique professional perspective while maintaining an active curiosity and actively soliciting the same from other team members. Opportunities for frequent, productive dialogue between team members facilitate the development of a common sense of purpose, which enables them to strategically leverage their unique professional and personal contributions. Interprofessional dialogue, at its most productive, is the art of thinking together and embracing different points of view (Isaacs, 1999).

Wheatley (2005) offers some provocative questions that can guide dialogue and help a healthcare team to define a unique, interdisciplinary culture that is strengthened by the diversity of its disciplinary parts. The questions are:

- Who are we?
- What matters?
- What do people talk about and where do they spend their energy?
- What topics generate the most energy—positive or negative?
- What issues do people talk about most?
- What stories do they tell over and over?
- Is it possible to develop a sense of shared purpose without denying our diversity?
- Are there ways that we develop a shared sense of what is significant without forcing people to accept someone else's viewpoint?

The interprofessional healthcare team is, at its best, a community of practice—a community of practice that is sustained by ongoing and productive dialogue and continuous learning. Wenger (2006) describes a community of practice as "a group of people who share a concern or passion for something they do and learn how to do it better as they interact regularly" (p. 1).

There are three distinguishing features of a community of practice. They are shared interest; engagement in information-sharing activities; and a development of shared resources such as experience, stories, and strategies for problem solving that facilitate the learning of all participants—a shared practice. The conceptualization of the interprofessional healthcare team as a community of practice brings into high relief the basic values of patient- and relationship-centered practice that defines a collaborative interdisciplinary culture. Wenger (2006) notes a variety of activities that can help to span disciplinary boundaries and facilitate the development of a community of practice and a culture of collaboration. The examples in **Table 8-1** show how these activities can be used to support a collaborative interdisciplinary culture.

Culture varies with the team and organization and is most aptly explained through the stories that are told by the members of the culture. It is the tone of the day-to-day interactions that gives us an insight into the web of values and behaviors that

TABLE 8-1 Examples of Boundary-Spanning Activities That Support a Collaborative Culture

Problem solving:

Can we get together to design a tool to evaluate the effectiveness of our caregiver training program?

Requests for information:

Where can I find the appropriate reimbursement codes for this diagnosis?

Seeking experience:

Has anyone dealt with a bilateral amputee with dementia?

Reusing assets:

I have a protocol that I have used with care givers of persons with dementia. I can help you adapt it for use on your unit.

(continues)

TABLE 8-1 Examples of Boundary-Spanning Activities That Support a
Collaborative Culture *(Continued)*

Coordination and Synergy:
Can we collaborate on our patient education process and save time and resources?
Documentation projects:
What are some examples of best practice? What went right? How can we make that the norm?
Visits:
Can we sit in on your in-service program? We think we may have similar needs.
Mapping knowledge and identifying gaps:
What information are we lacking for patients with left ventricular assist devices? We provide excellent cardiac rehabilitation but this is a new patient group for us. What other individuals/groups should we connect with?

Adapted from: Wenger (2006) Communities of Practice: a brief introduction.
http://www.ewenger.com/theory

comprise a culture. The following profiles are based on interviews
with health professional leaders and provide real-world perspectives on interprofessional teams.

Dr. Mary Sinnott, PT, DPT

Dr. Mary Sinnott is currently an assistant professor and director of the Doctor of Physical Therapy Program (DPT) at Temple
University, Philadelphia, Pennsylvania. Prior to coming to Temple
University, Dr. Sinnott was the director of physical therapy at
Thomas Jefferson Hospital in Philadelphia. In addition to her faculty and educational administration roles, she currently is actively
engaged in clinical practice at Temple University Hospital and is
a member of the American Physical Therapy Association board
of directors.

ON INTERPROFESSIONAL TEAMS

I use the term *interprofessional* rather than *interdisciplinary*
team. A report by the Institute of Medicine recommended the

use of *interprofessional* partly in an attempt to speak to physicians. Many physicians interpreted the term *interdisciplinary* to mean different disciplines within medicine; i.e., cardiology versus dermatology. To me, an interprofessional team is one that incorporates all of the disciplines and professions required to move a client to achieve their goals. The team may be composed of any number of professions; e.g. MD, nursing, PT, OT, respiratory therapy, etc. This diversity and representation of different viewpoints makes it possible for the team to work toward the patient's goals and achieve what they want to achieve. To use a metaphor, an interprofessional team is like a 12-lead EKG. Much like a 12-lead EKG gives you 12 views of the heart, you get many different views of a case.

I feel that there are a number of things that are critical to an effective interprofessional team—a culture of trust, a culture of open communication, a focus on the patient, leaving egos at the door, and having the right people on the team.

When I reflect on successful interprofessional teams that I have been a part of, the relationships and the time that we spent building relationships was key. It was not just relationship building through the institutional structure. You cannot force relationships. It happened first of all with an understanding and consensus of what the patient had to accomplish. As a physical therapist, I do not have goals. There are no PT goals; the patient has goals. I ask myself these questions: "What can I as a PT contribute to the patient's goals?" "How are others on the team looking at the goals?" In this ongoing conversation, you learn the perspectives of the other team members, and roles become clear. As a team you can answer the ongoing question, "Who on the team can best address the issues that are important to this patient?"

Each team is unique to the setting or to an individual patient's needs. It is not enough to say, "I know what OT is." The question is, "What is the role of OT in this particular patient's care?" The more I know about how you practice as a profession, the better teammates we can be. I know that you are an occupational therapist, so I will share with you that I have had the privilege of working with three outstanding OTs. They taught me a great deal and have, for me, set the standard for OT practice.

Formal team meetings contributed to the success of the team. But they were only one part of the success. It depended on who was leading the meeting and the "voice" of the leader. It was more of the informal interaction. The most productive interactions were not even in the formal team meetings but when I was cotreating with someone, or I would ask for advice. For example, I would ask the speech-language pathologist for suggestions on how to best communicate with a patient who was exhibiting expressive aphasia outside of formal meetings. This kind of consultation and help would not take place in the formal team meeting.

Team members were very comfortable with this combination of formal and informal structure. You also knew when someone was not a fit for the team because no one went to them for help. In this successful experience we left our egos at the door. There is a difference between confidence and ego. We were confident professionals. We were confident enough to check our egos and interact as a team.

In my experience, one of the stumbling blocks to a successful team is ego. Ego gets in the way of communication and collaboration. It puts blinders on people. They do not see the need to view the case in a different way. To go back to my metaphor, they are like a one-lead EKG. In summary, "None of us is as smart as all of us."

ON BUILDING A COLLABORATIVE CULTURE

Culture is the last and hardest thing to change in order for an organization to be successful. You can begin by building trust and honest communication. In an atmosphere of trust and honest communication, you can look for innovative solutions to problems and not assign blame. With trust, people know what your institutional motives are.

If I think about the roles that I play as a leader, these come to mind: consensus builder for a majority, not unanimity; negotiator; communicator; trust builder, to earn people's trust and ensure that they could trust me. These roles are linked to my leadership philosophy. I have thought quite a bit about my philosophy, and the foundation of it is to take care of relationships.

As a leader, you really don't achieve anything on your own. You need to take care of relationships so you can take care of business. As both a team member as well as a leader, developing and maintaining relationships is day-to-day work that ultimately makes you successful.

Both a team leader and the members have to have a clear vision of the role of the individual versus the responsibility of the team as a whole. Overarching is the role of a professional and the responsibilities and behaviors of a professional. If there is a professional atmosphere it sets up an expectation for professionalism. To me, professionalism requires interdependence. There is no room for dependence or independence. A leader can foster interdependence by modeling interdependence.

The culture of a setting is critical. When I counsel students, I always speak to the culture of a setting. Young professionals frequently underestimate the importance of organizational culture on their ability to be successful. They know very quickly if it is a good fit or if it is not a fit. If the setting is not a good fit they may feel trapped. In addition to being successful, every healthcare professional wants to feel proud of what they are doing.

As a leader, you need to have a clear idea of your culture and what behaviors you will and will not tolerate. I try to recruit people who are a good fit by asking questions about who prospective employees are as people. I am not hiring their credentials or diploma, I am hiring the person. The leader must know the culture and ask pointed questions to evaluate the fit. If people don't fit a culture or mission, it makes it harder to achieve your institutional goals.

The culture of an organization can support teams by demanding respect. Each member of the team is respected and respects their colleagues. How an institution treats people is key. Commitment to mission is another important foundation. An institution can live its mission by providing resources for the team, living a mission—not just having a mission on paper—and being truly patient or client centered.

Leaders can support the institutional culture through frequent environmental analysis. By this I mean talking to everyone in the system. Get out of the office and be proactive. Continually analyze systems to ensure that they facilitate goal attainment and again, ensure open lines of communication. If the information stops flowing in an organization, it stops at the weak link.

Exemplary institutional cultures engage in modeling more than training. In my experience, currently and in the past, individuals were chosen for leadership development training. Managers were selected for the training and the expectation was that the concepts would filter down to other levels of the organization. I personally feel that you can always learn new leadership skills, and with increased skills you understand the importance of being even more interdependent.

A STORY OF A SUCCESSFUL TEAM

I recently received a physical therapy consult for a 68-year-old woman who was admitted to the hospital from home. The chart said that she was independent at home but had recently experienced a change in her mental status. It was the end of the day and the physicians were planning for her discharge that day. One might question the need for a physical therapy consult for a patient with mental status changes, but in this facility, a PT consult was standard procedure prior to discharge. The referral indicated that the patient was medically stable. I went to the patient's room and found a resident and medical student managing the case. I introduced myself as the physical therapist and questioned the resident about the case. The resident did not appear to have a clear perspective on the patient's functional level. In the room I met the patient and her family. Her daughter was crying. In a conversation away from the patient, the daughter said emphatically, "Mom cannot go home!" The daughter reported that her mother could not go home because she had started to fall as a result of her rapidly deteriorating mental status. The daughter could not continue to care for her mother. She had two small children, was working full time and had recently been divorced. She would come home and find her mom on the floor! As I assessed the patient, I demonstrated and explained to the resident and medical student. Her balance was horrific! She was clearly not safe! The decision was made that she could not go home. She was a clear fall risk. I admit that I also made an assumption about the patient's level of function based on the referral information. I went to the room thinking that PT would not be indicated and found that this patient clearly needed an aggressive PT program. I was able to convey that to the physician. Working together (and in consultation with the attending physician), the resident, the daughter, and I were able to stop an unsafe discharge. To this day when the resident sees me in the hospital, he comes up to me. In this case, an intelligent conversation between disciplines led to a positive patient outcome. As I reflect on this case I feel that it was successful because I introduced myself to the resident, was clear about what I had to offer as a physical therapist, and engaged the physician and the family (most importantly, the daughter) into an interprofessional conversation that focused on the needs of the patient. And, as I said, the resident learned the benefits of interprofessional collaboration and specifically about the values of ordering a PT screening prior to discharge.

PERSPECTIVES ON THE FUTURE OF TEAMS IN HEALTH CARE

I feel that there is a positive shift on the importance of healthcare teams that continues to occur. The Institute of Medicine has made a strong case for the development of interprofessional teams. A number of health professions currently have written into their accreditation standards that students must be educated in teamwork. New physicians in all specialties demonstrate a greater willingness to be interdependent. This, I feel, is a culture shift in the practice of medicine. This culture shift will have a positive impact on the structure of teams and shared leadership. When designing the treatment plan for a specific patient, physicians will now ask, "Tell me what you think (as a PT)."

Dr. Tim Fox, PT, DPT, GCS, and Dr. Robyn Kurilko, PT, DPT

Dr. Tim Fox is the founder and chief executive officer (CEO) of Fox Rehabilitation. Dr. Robyn Kurilko is the executive vice president of clinical operations of Fox Rehabilitation. Founded in

1998, Fox Rehabilitation is a high-growth entrepreneurial private practice of full-time physical, occupational, and speech therapists, which is headquartered in Cherry Hill, New Jersey. Fox Rehabilitation was built on the foundation of geriatric House Calls, providing innovative home-based services to community-dwelling seniors. Diversification strategies have included outpatient clinics, skilled nursing rehabilitation, and pediatric centers. Fox Rehabilitation clinicians provide clinically excellent care and are given the autonomy they need to rehabilitate lives through evidence-based interventions.

ON INTERPROFESSIONAL TEAMS

We gave considerable thought to how the interprofessional team concept is reflected at Fox. I remember 15 years ago, when I worked in the rehab department of an acute care hospital, it was different than it is in House Calls. In acute rehab, every member of the team gathered around the patient's bed and discussed the case before moving to the next bed. That model is clearly not what we see in our practice!

From our perspective, in House Calls, private practice, our formal interprofessional team is very limited. We typically treat with a referral from a physician, make a phone call to schedule an appointment, and knock on the patient's door. Upon the conclusion of my initial exam, I generally contact my OT colleagues and initiate the dialogue, share data and perspectives, and begin to develop a plan. It is my responsibility to identify the team members, initiate communication, and coordinate the care; otherwise I will be providing care in a vacuum.

At Fox, a key member of the team is the caregiver. We cannot overlook the contribution of the caregiver or family in a geriatric practice. We often see spouses or other family members in the midst of a dramatic role change or role shift. In one ED (emergency department) visit, family members can transition from being a spouse or daughter immediately to a caregiver.

When we examine the successful teams that we have been a part of, they have three important characteristics in common. Members engage in consistent communication; members have a shared value of the services that they are providing; and all members demonstrate a sincere commitment to the patient and their colleagues. In House Calls, our clinicians have a very strong sense of team, but they need to construct the team specifically for each client.

Significant barriers to the sense of teamspirit we encounter are unclear expectations. Many times these unclear expectations start with the patient. Therapy is tough, and we as clinicians need to dose the intensity and frequency of treatment properly to ensure that the physiological change takes place. Physiological change is needed to support function. Patients need to understand and value the treatment and connect the link between progress in therapy, improved function, and independence and their ability to remain at home safely. Professionals need to encourage this understanding for the patient and family, to ensure active participation as important members of the treatment team.

ON BUILDING A COLLABORATIVE CULTURE

Fox Rehabilitation is not a traditional small business. I prefer to classify it as a high-growth, entrepreneurial private practice. We make significant clinical contributions to the populations that we serve. As the CEO, I have to look far beyond the horizon. The decisions that I make today will impact us far into the future.

Strong organizations stay true to their mission. Our mission believes in the strength of people. At Fox, our staff comes first. People ask, "How can that happen?" Happy, well-trained clinicians make good health care. It's really quite simple. If clinicians are respected, excited about coming to work, are well trained, and have excellent clinical skills, excellent patient care falls right into place.

There are a number of things that we do as a practice to facilitate and build an interprofessional culture—we expect it. In the teaching and training of our staff, we offer a balance of interprofessional and discipline-specific educational opportunities to support professional development.

Our clinicians continually reinforce our culture of attaining the highest level of clinical excellence possible from the moment our clinicians join our practice. Our commitment is demonstrated by a five-day orientation for new clinicians.

Monthly staff meetings are interprofessional and have a clinical focus such as review of function outcome measures, focus on evidence treatment techniques, and journal review.

Our clinical leadership is represented by occupational therapists, physical therapists, and speech-language pathologists who are provided the tools they need to support every clinician in their region as it relates to their documentation skills, clinically excellent care, and professional development.

A STORY OF A SUCCESSFUL TEAM

An interprofessional approach to patient care has been demonstrated to result in improved patient outcomes, reduced recidivism, and fewer overall healthcare dollars. In many cases, physical therapists in the home setting coordinate referrals to other skilled rehabilitation professionals. The following case study describes the coordination of an interdisciplinary team during a Medicare Part B House Calls visit.

ON THE FUTURE OF TEAMS IN HEALTH CARE

The research is clear from entities such as the Pew Foundation and the Institute of Medicine that interprofessional collaboration in healthcare leads to better patient outcomes.

I stay current on the literature related to pending changes in policy and regulation associated with health policy, regulation, and healthcare reform. As a leader of a progressive and innovative healthcare practice, it is always critical to collect as much data on a given topic as possible. Once you are certain you have the best and most stable data, you then layer in the vision, mission, culture, and a great deal of foresight. Notwithstanding the uncertainty and outcomes associated with healthcare reform, one thing will be certain. Professionals will need to increase the need to communicate more effectively and efficiently. The wise and thoughtful use of secure technology should facilitate such dialogues, ultimately improving interdisciplinary communication and patient wellbeing.

CASE STORY

A 72-year-old male presented 18 months following a left cerebral vascular attack (CVA). He had not received skilled rehabilitation intervention since a brief episode of home care following discharge from a skilled rehab facility. The referral for physical therapy was initiated by a visiting physician at the request of the patient's caregiver. The caregiver noticed difficulty with bed mobility and was concerned about the patient's lack of activity and decreased ability to perform activities of daily living (ADLs). Initial physical therapy findings included right hemiplegia, right upper extremity contracture, gross left-sided weakness, and difficulty with transfers. Additional findings included dysphagia, expressive aphasia, dependent ADLs, and suspected depression. The physical therapist contacted the visiting physician and recommended additional referrals to occupational and speech-language pathology services to address these deficits. In addition, the physical therapist assisted in coordinating the referral process.

In this case, the interprofessional rehabilitation team was coordinated by the initial treating physical therapist. Communication was maintained throughout the duration of care between the patient, caregiver, visiting physician, occupational therapist, speech-language pathologist, and physical therapist. Goals were created to address the needs and wants of the patient and caregiver. In this interprofessional team approach, each discipline was able to effectively address the patient's impairments. The patient's pathological condition and pharmacologic management were addressed by the visiting physician; strengthening, flexibility, and aerobic capacity were treated by the physical therapist; cognition, swallowing, and speech were addressed by the speech-language pathologist and the ADLs were treated by the occupational therapist. Positive outcomes were achieved by working together through an interprofessional coordinated care team, led by the physical therapist.

Sue Carol Verrillo, RN, MSN

Sue Carol Verrillo is the nurse manager of the Comprehensive Integrated Inpatient Rehabilitation program, Department of Physical Medicine and Rehabilitation, at The Johns Hopkins Hospital in Baltimore, Maryland. The services that are provided on this unit include physical therapy, occupational therapy, speech and language therapy, psychology, rehabilitative nursing, social services, therapeutic nutritional and dietary services, therapeutic recreation, prosthetics and orthotics prescription and fitting, pharmacist counseling, and respiratory therapy.

ON INTERPROFESSIONAL TEAMS

On a day-to-day basis, I see an interprofessional team that is working. A team is working when each of the members, nurses, therapists, physicians, social workers, psychologists, etc., feel free to bring up issues that are important to a patient. I can give you a recent example. We had a patient on the unit who was very complicated medically. An occupational therapist was seeing the patient in the morning for ADLs. The OT discovered that the patient's mother (whom she lived with) was ill herself and had a 24-hour caregiver. So the situation now was that a patient with a serious medical need was scheduled to go home with a parent who would not be able to care for her. This was clearly an unsafe discharge. The situation was presented to the interprofessional team; and a new plan needed to be developed. This level of commitment to the patient and the team is needed to ensure that the proper resources are in place for the best and safest discharge.

On a well-functioning interprofessional team, the boundaries of the disciplines dissolve, and everyone works together for the benefit of the patient. Effective teams require the flow of communication among and between the disciplines. It is about creating a total picture of the patient. It requires that all team members be patient centered and holistic.

I feel that one key to the development and functioning of interprofessifonal teams lies in empowerment by the leadership. The leadership empowers the team by giving them the tools, training, and an understanding of what patient-centered care looks like. Leadership then models effective teamwork on a day-by-day basis in multiple circumstances.

As I said before, teams need specific tools and training to make them the best they can be. A key blockage to effective interprofessional communication—that one needs to be aware of and guard against—is day-to-day busyness. It creeps in. When staff are up to their eyeballs with discipline-specific tasks that they must attend to, communication then becomes the most vulnerable to being compromised. For example, if a patient is exhibiting medical complications and the nurses are monitoring vital functions and medication levels and only communicating with the attending physician, then the opportunity to communicate what is happening with that patient to the rest of the team may be lost. The disciplines then can easily retreat into their silos. It is precisely at these crucial times, when the patient's care is the most complicated—that interprofessional communication is key.

ON BUILDING A COLLABORATIVE CULTURE

Communication and teamwork techniques need ongoing training. Without well-planned training, the team does not work well, and there is a tendency for professionals to revert back into previously learned modes of communication that are less effective and may compromise team functioning. If, for example, the physical therapist only reports on the patient's transfer status, but doesn't mention that the patient told them during the session that their spouse just lost their job, necessitating a social work consult, it is limiting and delays the progress of the whole team being able to address the identified need. If team members are encouraged to speak up, it becomes the team standard and the culture of the team. New members absorb this culture informally (by seeing it modeled) and formally (by attending training sessions), and it becomes self-perpetuating. I have seen that evolve with our own team.

When new employees are brought aboard, they are oriented to our standards and expectations of teamwork and communication through an eight-hour workshop. If staffing allows for all new staff to be together, we break it up into sets of sessions that each focus on specific communication techniques and teamwork principles. This has worked well for us. Staff participates in active sessions where they learn specific communication strategies involving various other disciplines, to see everyday issues from other perspectives. It gets staff up to speed with what we expect. It also empowers them to advocate for their patients and to speak up to other healthcare providers. We incorporate examples from our own unit to demonstrate the benefits of good teamwork and communication as well as the problems that can occur when communication and teamwork are lacking. We also reinforce that their input is highly valued.

We have developed an interprofessional communication system here that grew out of our teamwork and communication classes, called Report Doc. All professionals for the shift-to-shift handoff use it. We now know everything about the patient, from the perspectives of multiple disciplines, such as how they did in therapy, if there was a change in their diet (because they passed their swallow study), or a change in the amount of pain medicine that they require. For example, if the psychologist has determined that a particular patient does best if they are presented with only two choices per task, they would note this and team members could incorporate this strategy into their treatment sessions. Or, if PT notes that the patient's ability to transfer has improved and they now require only minimal assistance, nursing uses this information to assign staff for the next shift.

This reporting system also has a column for anticipated needs and factors to watch for. Each team member is able to see the to-do list of his or her colleagues and again the communication is enhanced.

Earlier I alluded to busyness as being a block to good teamwork. I feel, as a leader, it is my role to make sure that busyness does not creep in and impede the overall team function. I am vigilant and listen to end-of-shift reports to be sure that interdisciplinary communication is happening. Just this morning I encouraged a nurse to call a wound care specialist to address an urgent wound issue noted. Again, the threat is that communication will begin to shut down just when the complexity of the patient care requires it most.

A STORY OF A SUCCESSFUL TEAM

I have a story that is different in that it is a story of teamwork that did not take place on my unit. I am a knowledge specialist for the Johns Hopkins Institute of Nursing. The institute provides training for nurses from other countries either in their own institutions or here at the Johns Hopkins Hospital. On our unit we frequently have nurses visiting who work in rehabilitation or other specialties in their home countries. They are very interested in our systems and how we deliver care. I was approached by the Johns Hopkins Institute of Nursing to do a live videoconference on evidence-based practice for nurses in the United Arab Emirates. I had to develop the content—using the Johns Hopkins model of evidence-based practice, in conjunction with the Johns Hopkins Institute of Nursing. Then IT (information technology), the Johns Hopkins Institute liaison, and I had to collaborate, even though we had never worked together before, on the technical aspects of making sure the live video feed was working, in order for the teaching to be successful. There was a 12-hour time difference and 200 nurses at the other end of the connection! There were a few glitches, but it went very well. As I reflect on this experience, I realize it was very different for me. It was exciting but scary at the same time. I had to trust these professionals. I have no knowledge of how to set up a video conference! I was not in control of the situation. This made it more critical that we functioned as a team. We moved forward to success. You describe it as "not knowing" or "negative capability." That is what I experienced! As I think about it now, every day on an interprofessional team, very capable people who need to trust the capabilities of each other surround us.

ON THE FUTURE OF TEAMS IN HEALTH CARE

In the future, we will need to continue to stay ahead of communication issues. As patient care becomes more complex, there will be a need for even more interprofessional interaction. There are communication challenges that we face every day. One that I think of is the increased use of computers in health care. We have always heard that computers would make patient care easier. In my experience, the use of computers has made health care more accessible but also more complicated. We as leaders need to be aware of the hidden costs of computerization to the bedside healthcare provider. We need to continue to focus on the current concepts of working smarter, not harder. I have an example.

When residents begin, they are trained early in their orientation to the computer system on the unit. However, they may not actually rotate onto the unit for six months. By this time, they have forgotten the intricacies of the computer's order system functionalities. As a result, incorrect orders are frequently entered into the electronic record. The nursing staff, out of concern for patient safety, completes a thorough admission order reconciliation to the discharge worksheet and discharge summary and bring the discrepancies to the attention of the on-call resident. This takes significant time away from patient care and other important duties for both the physician and nurse, and it negatively impacts staff and physician morale. This problem is being zealously addressed through leadership attention, lean sigma, IT, and resident/nursing input to design a robust and effective solution. In short, I feel that healthcare teams are currently challenged not only to solve more complex clinical problems of patients, but also solve more complex system problems.

Dr. Emily Keshner, PT, EdD

Dr. Keshner is the professor and chair of the Department of Physical Therapy in the College of Health Professions and Social Work (CHPSW) at Temple University in Philadelphia, Pennsylvania, where she also serves as director of research strategy. Her research is focused on developing new treatment interventions that will effectively reduce instability and falls in aging and clinical populations. Her scientific work has taken an interprofessional approach, requiring the collaboration of physiologists, biomechanists, and bioengineers.

ON INTERPROFESSIONAL TEAMS

To me, a team is a group that is working toward a common goal or focus. I think I prefer focus because the goals for each team member may be different. I may have a goal for a patient to improve his ambulation, and you may have a goal of improving his community access. Both of us are focused on improving the patient's overall function. It allows each of us to focus on what we do best.

If we are going to have a truly operational healthcare system designed to help people with multiple problems—physical and psychological—we need all of the knowledge bases that are represented by different healthcare professionals talking to each other and working together. For example, if, as a PT, I can get someone to hold a spoon, they still cannot feed themselves if they have a swallowing problem. We need to begin the interprofessional process by identifying all of the difficulties we anticipate in a case and who is best suited to address each problem. The leader of the team should be the team member who is taking care of the primary issue that is being addressed at the moment.

One of the positive changes that I see developing is a shift in the assumption that the leader of the team is the physician. As the patient's needs change, the person leading the team shifts. The person who moves into this leadership position is the one who has the best perspective and understanding of the problem that is a priority at the moment. The leader may be the PT, speech-language pathologist, pharmacist, etc. The team must continue to make judgments to determine how they can address the multiple problems that are impeding a patient's function.

Blocks to team treatment can be summed up in one word—egos! It is not the only block but a major one. When you let your sense of self interfere with the end result of the team process, you are a blocker. Each person has to ask themselves "Do I want to be part of a team?"

Even in research, no system operates on its own. In the development of my research projects, I started reaching out to people in engineering to help me understand complex databases. I reached out to mathematicians to help me understand computational models. I brought in a biomechanist who had a better understanding of mechanics of motion. I brought my skills as a neuroscientist and my clinical point of view to the project. By assembling a team, we were able to ask more complicated questions. We focused on researching a question that would have practical implications.

In research, I see that people often "silo" themselves. They learn the skills of a single discipline. They try to solve all of the problems that they encounter through the knowledge base of that discipline. I find great value in multiple scientists working together. I have had the good fortune to be a part of many great teams made up of a diverse group of individuals who had a variety of perspectives. When I reflect on what has made them successful, these four factors come to mind: equanimity, open communication, common interests, and opportunities for personal development. The contribution of each member on the team was respected. Many times, I was a member of a team that was made up of clearly senior and junior members. This did not mean that the senior members had the final say. The communication was characterized by intellectual sharing and openness. There was an ongoing process of learning. It was not progressive learning; it is integrated learning where we are all learning at the same time and from each other.

In my capacity as an educator, I have also given a lot of thought to interprofessional education. To implement interprofessional education, barriers will need to be broken down. In the ideal, there would be a community of health care where, instead of each of the departments being housed on its own floor, faculty would be mixed in clusters that had common interests; e.g., a neuroscience cluster or an orthopedic cluster. Also, we need to offer courses that cross disciplines such as healthcare ethics or group processes. We should explore redesigning our curricula so that students from different disciplines would work on projects where they bring their unique skill set to the case. I know that we have been talking about interprofessional education for 40 years. Unfortunately, it continues to be a difficult concept to operationalize.

ON BUILDING A COLLABORATIVE CULTURE

From a research perspective, I have begun to look aggressively for funding sources for projects that have a broad impact on health. I am looking to develop projects that do not focus on one question only. Projects that may have a broader focus would be research that is directed at changing healthcare delivery models or modeling systems designed to deliver healthcare to underserved populations. This would provide me with the opportunity to pull team members from a number of disciplines who would be able to identify their contribution to such an interprofessional project.

I have also participated and organized social events that were designed to get researchers talking in a more informal way. We have had happy hours and also an event called research speed dating. During research speed dating, participants spoke for four minutes and then moved on to the next table. These affairs gave faculty an opportunity to interact with colleagues to see what their research interests were as well as get to know each other at a more personal level. It made it easier for them to reach out to each other. When opportunities came up for collaborative projects, they had a network.

From the academic perspective, what I would like to see is a change in the culture of curriculum. My hope is that professionals in the future will not have to work as hard when they are practicing to understand what others on the healthcare team do. I hope that the next generation of students will develop with the expectation that they have to know what a patient needs and collaborate with other professionals. We could potentially utilize the IOM recommendations for interprofessional education as standards to design an integrated curriculum.

Two factors that come into play as potential roadblocks in designing interprofessional experiences are funds and scheduling. A grant could help us design and examine interprofessional strategies. We also need to consider more creative uses of time. Scheduling is always an issue. Utilizing the summers or weekends or seminar formats may be a possibility.

A STORY OF A SUCCESSFUL TEAM

Last summer I was part of an exciting interprofessional project. I had secured a grant to support undergraduate students' research. I had six students from different majors ranging from computer science to kinesiology to psychology. I shared the grant with a faculty member from computer science. The research mentors in the project were also a diverse group—computer science, neuroscience, etc. We developed five projects that provided the students opportunities to utilize their special skills. For example, the computer science students developed the programs that we needed. The psychology and kinesiology students collected data using the programs developed by the computer science students. Much of the success of the program, I feel, was in the atmosphere that we created. Both my coinvestigator and I are very enthusiastic people and understood what we were trying to accomplish. He had the role of supporting the technology in the laboratory so that I could focus on the science. I know that I depended on his technological skills. We engaged in respectful sharing. We had weekly lab meetings where we shared both progress and problems. A process of group problem solving addressed problems; we were a team. At the conclusion of the grant, students were required to reflect on the experience. One student wrote, "Everybody should have this experience. It was the best experience of my education." Further evidence of the success of this team experience is the fact that two of the projects are still running and three students registered for independent studies this year in order to continue working in the lab.

ON THE FUTURE OF TEAMS IN HEALTH CARE

As we move to more of an interprofessional focus, we cannot forget the human factor. Even if we say that we are dedicated team members and dedicated to solving common problems, we all have our own personal need to excel. We cannot lose our own identity. The team cannot become an amorphous group defined only by the whole.

John J. Kirby, OTR/L, MBA

John Kirby started his career as an occupational therapist in the specialty of hand therapy before moving into the acute care hospital environment and then eventually into hospital administration serving as a physician liaison and service line manager developing significant product lines for hospitals, which included a stroke center, orthopedic center of excellence in partnership with the a large private orthopedic group, and expansion of surgical services (vascular, general, and retinal). Eventually, he was recruited to the position of vice president of clinical operations, chief operating officer and then chief executive officer of the Pottstown Memorial Medical Center in Pottstown, Pennsylvania. He currently serves as associate executive director of operations at the Hospital of the University of Pennsylvania in Philadelphia.

ON INTERPROFESSIONAL TEAMS

I define interprofessional within the context of the program or the project that is being worked on. As a leader, you want to be sure that everyone who needs to be involved with the patient is there. I would say that we put the patient in the center of a circle and then determine who the key personnel are who can deliver the quality of care that we expect. That is your team.

I have learned that many times, smaller teams are better. I had the opportunity to work with a junior executive who was assigned to a project. In follow-ups, it became apparent to me that this team was not effective. There were too many people involved. They were not well organized. There was dissention in the team and they were not meeting deadlines. As I reflect on it, the problem may have been a combination of the level of team development and weak leadership. The structure of a team is key and needs to be a match for the project.

One of the most damaging blocks to team development and function is when members feel like they do not have a voice. Feeling like they are not really a team with decision-making power or the ability to give input into a project impedes any type of team function. Too much direction from upper level leadership as to what they expect and how it must be done interrupts a legitimate team process. Another block is a team that does not have a clear and shared vision. Communication is key and any block in the flow of information from top down or bottom up impedes team function. Finally, in hospitals and most large institutions, there is also the historical block. The "We tried that before" or "That has not worked in the past" comments are frequent blocks that are clearly designed to hijack change.

ON BUILDING A COLLABORATIVE CULTURE

In the current climate of health care, patients' perception of care and public reporting are very important. By public reporting, I mean factors, such as infection control rates, that are a matter of public record. Patients are also able to assess and compare hospitals on a number of reported measures and outcome data. For hospitals, like the community hospitals where I have worked in the past, this is important. We used these metrics every day. Behind each of these metrics is a hospital system or program. For example, a community hospital where I worked as an administrator had an active emergency room. People from the communities in our service area depended on the emergency room for care. If a patient comes into an emergency room and waits for hours because you do not have the personnel in place or there are no beds, you are saying, "You are not important to us." For example, we had a goal that no one would wait more than 22 minutes before being seen by a physician. Behind all of these successful metrics were team initiatives.

To me, as a leader, there are two important components to creating an interprofessional culture. Creating and sustaining this culture requires a combination of respect and accountability. You must model and demand that team members treat each other with respect. The leader must constantly assess the level of engagement of each team member. I feel that the effective leaders stay out of the way of the productive team members and work with the marginal team members one-to-one until they also are functioning as productive colleagues.

A STORY OF A SUCCESSFUL TEAM

The hospital that I was affiliated with made the decision to hire a vascular surgeon. State data showed that patients had been leaving our service area to get vascular procedures. In hiring a surgeon to lead the program, we looked for someone who shared our vision and had a plan on how to move that vision forward. We hired an MD who had a vision that was compatible with ours. This included a surgery program, a wound care program, a surgery center that would offer minimally invasive procedures, and a vein program. We were planning a full complement of services. I convened a team representing all of the persons that we would need to get the program running—OR staff, the MD, nursing, radiology, and the MD's office manager.

This was a very successful team. We had enough people but not too many. We had a very prescriptive process as to who was accountable for what and for reports that were due and the dates for delivery. The MD was at every meeting, and having him there reinforced the importance of this team and this project. This demonstrated clear leadership on his part.

This was an organization that had not invested in itself in a long time, so when the CEO made the commitment to the development of this program, the people in the organization were very excited. They saw this as an opportunity to grow and be proud. They recognized that the institution had a good vision. This was something that it had not had in a while. The communication was open and the engagement was exceptional. This was the first project that I had run myself. Having been a member of teams that were not successful, I vowed not to make those mistakes.

As the leader, I chose the team members. There were some that I knew needed to be approached one-to-one because I was afraid that they would not move at the pace that we needed to meet deadlines and move the project forward, and I needed to ensure their commitment. We were on a tight time frame. We did not want to lose the MD, and the institution was investing a lot of resources into the project. I energized and built enthusiasm by modeling excitement. I appealed to their pride in the hospital and the community by emphasizing that this project was allowing us to compete with the top hospitals in our service area. I also made sure that the team knew that I was not being micromanaged. I had the confidence and support of upper level leadership. The CEO formally and informally recognized and praised the work of the group.

The team kept rolling. They met deadlines. I gave them an opportunity to come to me to vent if they felt frustrated for any reason. I did not want anyone to feel frustrated or, as I say, "get plaque in their arteries!" For the most part, they recognized that the hospital's success was their success.

The conversation was open and direct. Conversations occurred at the formal meetings and outside of the meetings. Members assumed the role of leader in the areas that they were responsible for. Again, I want to emphasize that the MD worked diligently outside of the formal meetings. He deferred to the expertise of others in the group and approached the project from the perspective of evidence-based medicine. We structured the meetings around a live document that organized the project. This guiding document kept us moving, making decisions and meeting deadlines. To me, a meeting is where decisions are made and processes are approved. Much of the work is done outside of the meetings. That is my style. The document that we created is really a picture of the team and its activity. I also utilize a scoring grid that provides an opportunity for the team members to assess themselves.

The program and center opened on time and on target. It was very successful. As I reflect on it, this team was somewhat of an incubator for leadership development. Many of the members of that team are no longer with the hospital. They have moved to other, more administrative positions in hospitals and healthcare systems in the city. I am very proud of that and hope that this experience played a part in their success.

As a postscript, leading this project for me was an important lesson in succession planning. After the MD who founded the program left the hospital, the program floundered. It was a learning experience for me to be sure that in the future, when faced with such a large and extensive and expensive project, I built a leadership succession plan with a second tier of personnel. In this case, the inclusion of a junior-level MD on the team would have facilitated the sustainability of the team and the program.

ON THE FUTURE OF TEAMS IN HEALTH CARE

I believe that the best teams are smaller teams. I construct teams with key people and then bring in others when they are needed for specific tasks. You start with a core team and expand the membership when it is needed. This type of flexible approach has been very effective for me.

Rebecca Austill-Clausen, MS, OTR/L, FAOTA

Rebecca "Becky" Austill-Clausen, MS, OTR/L, FAOTA, is the president and owner of Austill's Rehabilitation Services, Inc., which was founded in 1984. Today, the company is a group of over 300 experienced occupational therapy practitioners, physical therapy practitioners, and speech-language clinicians. The company provides services to educational programs and healthcare communities throughout the Pennsylvania and Delaware Valley region. Austill's mission is to provide high-quality, cost-effective educational and rehabilitative services to pediatric and adult clients and agencies while simultaneously providing a stimulating and supportive environment for their family of therapists.

ON INTERPROFESSIONAL TEAMS

At Austill's, the core of our interdisciplinary team is comprised of occupational therapists, physical therapists, and speech-language clinicians. However, in the practice areas that we serve, the team expands. For example, in our school-based practice, the team includes teachers, principals, parents, and support services.

Austill's is organized by geographical regions. Each of the regions has a lead coordinator. The lead coordinator may be an occupational therapist, a physical therapist, or a speech-language pathologist. In this organizational structure, each therapist has a lead coordinator. The lead coordinator may or may not represent the same discipline. For example, an occupational therapist may report to a lead coordinator who is a physical therapist. There has never been a problem with this interprofessional reporting. If a therapist has a specific clinical question, he or she is referred to a lead coordinator who represents the same discipline. With this structure, we assure that each therapist is supported both administratively and clinically.

I feel that one of the biggest blocks to interprofessional teamwork is fear of the unknown. Fear of competition, fear of job loss, fear of the future. Yes, I think that fear is a huge block. I believe we can counteract fear through a combination of respect and confidence. By this I mean respect for each team member's specialty, respect for each member's position, education and training, and clinical expertise. In addition, all team members must feel confident and be comfortable with themselves, their skills, their professional identities, and their values. The combination of respect and confidence can diminish fear.

ON BUILDING A COLLABORATIVE CULTURE

At Austill's, our goal is to provide high-quality, cost-effective services. Our therapists are at the core of our business. We have three constituencies—our therapists, our service contractors, and the clients that we treat. If the therapists are happy, then everyone wins. Each year we poll our therapists to get an idea of what is working for them and what is not. We are interested and concerned about the therapists, their lives, and their ability to care for their families. For example, a therapist may want to start working later in the day to accommodate a child's school schedule. We strive to facilitate all therapists working their ideal jobs. We empower our staff. While this strategy may seem soft to some, it has been very successful for us. We have a very low staff turnover and an extremely satisfied customer base. Austill's is growing and thriving!

We are committed to getting to know each of our therapists at a personal level. We are committed to having the right match of our employees. In order to demonstrate that they are a fit for Austill's, a prospective employee must be able to clearly articulate what he or she is looking for in a position—what makes him or her happy? In addition, candidates need to be friendly, self-assured, independent, and professional. At the foundation, they must respect themselves and the value of their profession.

I value personal relationships. This value is central to the mission and success of Austill's. It is reflected in all of my team and group experiences. If you get to know people at a deeper level, it opens new channels of communication.

I strive to create a positive climate and empowering atmosphere. I love people and I listen to my heart. I use an open communication style and give people permission to say what they want, and I listen. I hire managers who are also positive, respectful, good listeners, collaborative, and goal directed.

As a leader I believe in getting people together. I look for commonalities to build upon. I always make and distribute an agenda. At the beginning of each meeting I start with introductions. The introductions help establish each member as an individual with an identity beyond the profession that they represent. I follow introductions with a review of the agenda—everyone is given the opportunity to add items. The basic structure is in place to move goals forward. I work diligently to create an atmosphere where collaboration and consensus are the norms.

A STORY OF A SUCCESSFUL TEAM

I was a member of an interprofessional group that represented rehabilitation services in home care for the Joint Commission (formerly the Joint Commission on the Accreditation of Healthcare Organizations (JCAHO). The members of the group represented the American Occupational Therapy Association (AOTA), the American Physical Therapy Association (APTA), the American Speech and Hearing Association (ASHA) and three therapeutic recreation associations. There were18 group members in total. I was the team leader and the only one who had a voice and a vote at the Joint Commission meeting. It was important that I went to the Joint Commission meeting with a clear idea of the ideas and feelings of each of the associations that I represented. We would meet as a group the night before the Joint Commission meeting to discuss the issues and achieve consensus. Before the meeting, I distributed an agenda. Each of the group members worked with their disciplinary associations and constituents to be sure that they accurately represented the issues. We would meet and work through the issues until we achieved 100% consensus and were able to speak with one voice. I feel that this process worked because each of the members of the group respected each other. We listened to each other—actively listened—and each member came to the meeting prepared. The day after the rehabilitation meeting, I joined nursing, medicine, and a number of other professions (there were 30 representatives in total), for a full-day Joint Commission meeting. I was the only voice for rehabilitation in home care at the table. As a team, we successfully lobbied for rehabilitation in home care. I feel that we were successful because each of the group members came prepared, respected each other, listened, and were committed to achieving consensus. We worked as a team. We understood that we were more powerful as a group than each of us would be individually. There was no feeling of empire building.

When I am a member or the leader of a successful team I get excited! Building consensus by mobilizing a diversity of viewpoints can be both challenging and great fun! Setting a goal and seeing that goal met is thrilling.

ON THE FUTURE OF TEAMS IN HEALTH CARE

One big change that I see is that we are becoming so dependent on technology that communication is not face-to-face. For me, the challenge is to keep a very successful relationship-centered organization communicating and growing using technology in a user-friendly fashion. We have established some small learning communities within the regions that Austill's serves. We are developing online educational programs and utilize an extensive self-designed custom database to maximize communication and collaboration. We will continue to expand the use of technology to create additional learning community opportunities and facilitate personal interaction and interactive experiences.

REFLECTION: *Analyzing Team Cultures*

- What levels of culture (artifacts, espoused values, and basic assumptions) are reflected in these profiles?
- What characteristics of collaborative teams are in evidence?
- What characteristics of a community of practice are in evidence?
- What leadership behaviors were used to foster a collaborative environment?
- Can you see these characteristics and behaviors at work in your setting?
- What is your successful team story?

References

Anchor, S. (2012, January–February). Positive intelligence. *Harvard Business Review, 90*(1–2), 100–102.

Briskin, A., Erickson, S., Ott, J., & Callanan, T. (2009). *The power of collective wisdom and the trap of collective folly.* San Francisco, CA: Berrett-Koehler.

Fox, J. (2012, January–February). The economics of well-being. *Harvard Business Review, 90*(1–2), 79–83.

Frederickson, B. (2003, July–August). The value of positive emotions. *American Scientist, 91*, 330–335.

Frederickson, B. (2009). *Positivity.* New York, NY: Crown.

Institutes of Medicine. (2001). *Crossing the quality chasm: A new health system for the 21st Century.* Washington, DC: National Academy Press.

Institutes of Medicine. (2002). *Who will keep the public healthy? Educating public health.* Washington, DC: National Academy Press.

Institutes of Medicine. (2003). *Health professions education: A bridge to quality.* Washington, DC: National Academy Press

Isaacs, W. (1999). *Dialogue and the art of thinking together.* New York, NY: Doubleday.

McKee, A., Tilin, F., & Mason, D. (2009). Coaching from the inside: Building an internal group of emotionally intelligent coaches. *International Coaching Psychology Review, 4*(1), 35–46.

Pew Health Professions Commission. (1998). *Recreating health professional practice for a new century: The fourth report of the Pew Health Professions Commission.* San Francisco, CA: Pew Health Professions Commission.

Schein, E. H. (1986). *Organizational culture and leadership.* New York, NY: Jossey-Bass Publishing.

Spreier, S., Fontaine, M., & Malloy, R. (2006, June). Leadership run amok: The destructive potential of overachievers. *Harvard Business Review*, pp. 73–82.

Spreitzer, G., & Porath, C. (2012, January–February). Creating sustainable performance. *Harvard Business Review, 90*(1–2), 92–99.

Wenger, E. (2006). Communities of practice: A brief introduction. Retrieved from http://www.ewenger.com/theory

Wheatley, M. (2005). *Finding our way: Leadership for an uncertain time.* San Francisco, CA: Berrett-Koehler Publishers, Inc.

Wheatley, M. (2006). *Leadership and the new science: Discovering order in a chaotic world.* (3rd ed.). San Francisco, CA: Berrett-Koehler Publishers, Inc.

Whitney, D., Trosten-Bloom, A., & Radu, K. (2010). *Appreciative leadership: Focus on what works to drive winning performance.* New York, NY: McGraw-Hill.

World Health Organization (WHO). (2006). *The world health report 2006: Working together for health.* Geneva, Switzerland: The World Health Organization.

Zolno, S. (2007). Towards a healthy world: Meeting the challenges of the 21st century. *Linkage,* (34), 14.

CHAPTER **9**

Generative Practices

Learning Objectives

1. Use self-management to effect positive change in oneself and others.
2. Understand the importance of personal renewal.
3. Utilize language strategically to foster affirmative and productive team environments.
4. Match dialogue and discussion to the developmental needs of the team.
5. Understand the concept of appreciative inquiry.

Sustainable systems are resilient in the face of change. For the purposes of our discussion, generative practices are self-management and interactive strategies that empower individuals to believe in their value as agents of positive change and be proactive in facilitating that change. Garnering the power of the team is not unlike focusing on the strengths of an individual patient to achieve maximum function. It requires an analysis of the present level of function, an understanding of the ultimate goal of intervention, the therapeutic use of self, and the environment and the

187

active participation of the patient in order to achieve positive, sustainable change. The key to the sustainability of social systems like interprofessional healthcare teams is the consistent attention to the building of social capital—those systemic features that facilitate hope, vitality, self-efficacy, and relational coordination.

> Only when we join ourselves vitally with others in arrangements of shared power can we reach a new threshold of co-creativity and purpose. This kind of power can come only from individuals finding what is unique about themselves in order to best contribute to a healthier whole. Our differences and diversity makes the collective engine powerful. (Briskin et al, p. 90)

The emotional reality of a group, organization, or community is comprised of subtle, yet powerful underlying emotional currents that affect the overall climate, culture, and behavior of the group. Humans react, on a neurophysiological level, to the verbal and nonverbal cues that we receive and transmit to each other and can generally sense when someone is upset or excited (Ekman, 1997 Gottman, Levenson, & Woodin, 2001) This neural connectivity often facilitates emotional contagion—for good or ill—within groups. Another term for *positive emotional contagion* is *resonance*, while *dissonance* is synonymous with *destructive emotional contagion* (Ekman et al, 2003; Hatfield, Cacioppo, & Rapson, 1993; Strazdins, 2000). When a leader is perceived as angry, disrespectful, or unfair, these emotions are reciprocated and reverberate, creating a dissonant group culture (Boyatzis & McKee, 2005; Goleman, 2003).

The following are examples of practices that can facilitate the development and maintenance of a positive and sustainable team culture. The deliberate, conscious, and strategic use of interpersonal communication ensures that the limited time allotted to team interaction can be employed efficiently and effectively. These are practical methods by which organizations, groups, or individuals can foster a positive emotional climate and garner the infinite resources inherent to open systems and enable them to adapt and survive in an ever-changing world.

REFLECTION: *Responses to Nonverbal Clues*

Our bodies respond to our emotions in subtle and obvious ways. Facial expressions, tone of voice, changes in skin tone, and postural stances may be fleeting but important signs of the emotions that drive a person's behavior (Ekman, 2004; Hamm, Schupp, & Weike, 2003).

Think about a recent interaction that you have had.

- Describe the nonverbal clues that you picked up from the individual or individuals who were involved in the interaction.
- What did the clues tell you?
- How did those clues affect your behavior?

Heal Thyself: The Importance of Personal Renewal

In the high stakes healthcare arena, health professionals are often at the mercy of rapid change, needing to take big risks and often making what may feel like life-and-death decisions for themselves and their organizations. This means that health professionals are likely to be in a state of high arousal much of the time. Healthcare professionals may be more likely to suffer from the burnout and compassion fatigue that is associated with taking care of others and not taking care of themselves. Ironically, sacrificing self-care actually reduces the quality of care provided (Landro, 2012). This condition is magnified for leaders of healthcare teams who must navigate the myriad moral and financial challenges inherent to all healthcare organizations, who shoulder heavy responsibilities, and who are often distanced from people because of their position of power. It is not uncommon for leaders to succumb to the "sacrifice syndrome," which is described as a downward spiral of "internal disquiet, unrest and distress" (Boyatzis & McKee, 2005, p. 6). Unmitigated entanglement in such a destructive cycle wreaks havoc not only on the individual leader but on all of those with whom he or she comes in contact, resulting in poorly performing teams, high staff turnover, and poor outcomes.

In times of stress, the rational parts of the brain are likely to be affected by the more primitive, less rational parts of the brain.

As physical and psychological capacity is overloaded, individuals are likely to react with fight-or-flight responses, and the overall capacity to be creative, solve problems, and learn is compromised (Alvarez-Buylla & Temple, 1998; Dickerson & Kemeny, 2004) While the sympathetic nervous system (SNS) is responsible for the body's ability to react quickly and effectively to physical or emotional provocation, the parasympathetic nervous system (PSNS) is responsible for recovery from such excitement and for keeping the body on an even keel by lowering blood pressure and strengthening the immune system (Goleman, 2003; McEwen, 1998; Sapolsky, 2004). As a result, a sense of well-being is restored and maintained (Diener & Lucas, 2000; Diener, Suh, Lucas, & Smith, 1999). A person who feels this way is likely to be optimistic, less anxious and open to new learning and relationship building (Boyatzis & McKee, 2005).

REFLECTION: *Daily Self-Sustaining Behaviors*

The restorative nature of caring relationships, social networks, hope for the future, and mindful attention to the present stimulate PSNS activity and allow for intellectual, physical, and emotional renewal that is crucial to effective leadership and membership.

- What activities help you to feel energized and peaceful? (Walking, running, exercising, practicing yoga, meditating, painting, singing, dancing, etc.) Could you see yourself starting and/or ending each day this way?

- What are the situations that make you most angry or anxious? Can you imagine reacting to them in a different way? Next time, before you react, ask yourself: "In this situation—with these people—how could I move toward relationships?"

- How do you feel after you choose your reactions more mindfully or consciously? Are you more or less angry or anxious?

- What surprised you today at work? What did you learn? With regard to your work, what are you most grateful for? What do you hope to accomplish?

Affirmative Dialogue

In order to navigate the complexity of our existence, we create mental categories that aid in the processing of experiences, feelings, and our perception of people. The cognitive organization or "chunking" of this data enables us to expand our knowledge base, plan actions, predict outcomes, and learn from our experiences. As new information is processed, emotional memories are intertwined with the lived experience. At each step along the neurologic pathways, our primitive brain, in concert with our rational brain, make choices about what we believe we have seen, heard, and experienced (Dickerson & Kemeny, 2004). This cognitive process gives rise to the development of habits of thoughts and behavior that may be accurate, positive, and effective but may also be inaccurate, negative, and maladaptive (Langer & Imber, 1979). This is why "first impressions die hard." The research gives credence to this old adage and links emotions to in-the-moment behavior as well as to longer-term attitudes and judgments. For instance, we are often confused by, are mistrustful of, and have visceral reactions to persons who appear anxious, untrustworthy, or disrespectful. When we have experienced negative reactions to or from a person, we may develop a habitually defensive response to them rather than consciously choosing a response that is in tune with the current situation. We are likely to revert to mental and behavioral habits that may not be adapted to the situation at hand.

One of the manifestations of these behavioral habits is the tendency to interpret the behavior of others through the lens of

---

REFLECTION: *Shorthand Interpretations*

What are some of the shorthand interpretations you use in your team?

How might this facilitate or hinder your participation?

How might this facilitate or hinder the participation of others?

How might this facilitate of hinder the output of the team?

our own habits of thought or personal bias. For example, team members might think, "Oh, of course Jim would see the issue only in terms of money . . . He's a finance guy." Or, "Jane is always so resistant to anything new. We know what she will say so let's not even attempt to bring her in." Or, "Mike always speaks first and thinks later." While there might be some truth to these shorthand observations, they are also stereotypical and may not describe the individual's current perspective.

In the absence of mindful attention to the perspective of others, misperceptions can often devolve into polarization and disengagement of group members. If group members feel that they are misunderstood and marginalized, they are likely to react in defensive and unproductive ways. Conversely, affirming interactions acknowledge the members' ability to move the group in a positive direction. They feel valued and accepted and will be invested in the work and the outcome of the group. In a resonant team, Jim would be valued for his ability to analyze the most cost-effective way to approach a project, Jane would be valued for her historical knowledge and ability to critically examine issues and identify obstacles, and Mike would be valued for his spontaneity, enthusiasm, and creativity. Hope allows for the consideration and valuation of all of the group members' strengths, dreams, and visions for the future. These acts of affirmation trigger a sense of well-being that sets into motion a positive contagion. The result is a resonant group that is calm, elated, optimistic, energized, and prepared to leverage its collective strengths and transform vision into reality.

When routine interprofessional healthcare team meetings are characterized by positive interactive experiences, it is more likely that the teams will be able to respond in a rational, productive manner during times of stress. Conversations that are focused on the possibilities that each member offers for exemplary patient care are more likely to engage and sustain individuals, groups, and organizations and yield positive results in day-to-day as well as emergency situations (Ludema, 2001; Frederickson, 2003; Whitney, Trosten-Bloom & Radu, 2010). This concept is dramatically borne out by research on emergency room teams who had

EXAMPLES OF AFFIRMATIVE LANGUAGE

"We have every reason to be worried about this but maybe we can brainstorm some possible strategies to head this issue off."

"We seem to have spent the last 10 minutes talking about Sally and she is not even here. Maybe we can start to discuss how we can get this project done even if Sally cannot do what we think we want her to do."

"I think we all were disappointed that the last meeting with the patient didn't go the way we expected it to. I would like to discuss the lessons learned here so that we can do a better job next time. I know next time I will (. . . provide bilingual instructions, make sure we are clear about team member responsibilities, engage the caregivers in the discussions, etc.)."

favorable perceptions of their team dynamics and demonstrated lower mortality rates than their counterparts who viewed their teams unfavorably (Wheelan, Burchill, & Tilin, 2003).

The following are some examples of how one might handle a difficult situation by naming the behavior or issue that is of concern, acknowledging the negative feelings that it might engender and redirecting those feelings toward a positive action.

Reframing

The affirmative language used in the following box is an example of reframing or the strategic use of language to highlight the current situation from a new perspective with the intention of broadening the repertoire of behavioral choices. The three sample statements in the next box are fatalistic, dead-end streets that lead the speaker and the listener nowhere. The reframed options provide a more optimistic and proactive view of the same situations and are focused on shared values, goal attainment, and action and provide a variety of alternatives for action (Bandler & Grinder, 1975; Dilts, 1999; Hall & Bodenhammer, 2002).

REFRAMING EXAMPLES

1. Each health professional is trained differently. It is difficult to coordinate our intervention.

   Reframe:

   Having access to a variety of perspectives broadens the possibilities for innovative intervention strategies.

2. Finding a time when everyone can meet is too difficult.

   Reframe:

   Everyone's time is precious, and sharing information is crucial for good patient care. How can we use meeting time most effectively? When is the best time to meet? What are some other ways we can share information?

3. He didn't even respond when I gave my opinion . . . he just went on to the next person. It is obvious that he doesn't care about my opinion.

   Reframe:

   The meeting is almost over. It looks like he is trying to gather information from everyone while we are all together.

REFLECTION: *Strategic Use of Language*

We can use language strategically to facilitate a positive self-talk as well as positive team environment and stimulate positive action. Read the two sets of statements that follow. How do you feel after reading the first set of statements? How do you feel after reading the second set of statements?

STATEMENT SET I:

- He is disrespectful of the contributions of others.
- I don't know why I took on the coordination of this project. It is too much for me to do.
- She is absolutely crazy! Ignore her.
- He is too pushy and tries to insinuate himself into things that don't concern him.

STATEMENT SET II:

- He has a clear picture of what he thinks is best for the group. Could it be that he has a particular concern in mind that he has not shared with us?

- This is the kind of project that gets my creative juices flowing. I like doing the research and learning something new.

- Her view of reality is really vastly different than ours. We should discuss this further with her. Might there be a time/circumstance when that perspective could be instructive?

- He may seem pushy, but he really cares very deeply about them and wants to help in any way he can. Is his tendency to throw himself wholeheartedly into a task always a problem?

The Team as Learner

McMurtry (2007) views healthcare teams as "complex collective learners with knowledge emerging at the level of the team that exceeds the sum total of individual team members' knowledge" (p. 38). The institutionalization of opportunities for interprofessional healthcare teams to interact on a regular basis provides fertile ground for the development of shared perspectives (Clark, 2010). The following approaches employ a team's communication capacity to establish a collective identity based on shared values, interests, and strong relationships. As a result, curiosity, hope, and energy fuels ongoing learning and builds resiliency for all team members in the face of future change.

Interprofessional healthcare teams are often faced with complex problems. While there are diverse perspectives regarding possible solutions, the commonly held goal is the best possible patient outcome. An interesting five-stage model for approaching complex problem solving is proposed by Wheatley (2005). The stages are cooling/quieting, enriching, magnetizing, destroying, and acting. Respectively, the core behaviors/attitudes required for each stage are patience and curiosity, respect and clear thinking, generosity and humility, discipline and discernment, and cohesion and reflectivity. Structuring the physical environment as well as the discussion reflects the primary task of each stage.

Cooling/quieting: At this stage, each member of the team has an opportunity to share his or her perspective and understand how others perceive the problem. It is suggested that the team sits in a circle.

Discussion questions that might be appropriate for this stage would be:

- What is the aspect of this situation that you think is most important?
- What has been your experience in dealing with issues such as these?

Enriching: At this stage, it is suggested that the team sits in a square configuration so that sides or differences are amplified, and each side has an opportunity to provide a detailed rationale for its perspective. As a side is being presented, others listen. The result is a method for managing conflict and a more complete, collective understanding of all aspects of the issue. Paradoxically, the collective examination of differences of opinion often allow the team to emerge more unified and cohesively.

Discussion questions that might be appropriate for this stage would be:

- What new learning did you experience?
- How has your perspective changed?

Magnetizing: The trust and broadened perspective that is gained from passage through the other stages allows the development of strong interpersonal relationships, collective acceptance that there is not one best way, and a willingness to accept that there may be additional viewpoints that the team has yet to discover. A half-circle seating arrangement facing an open area echoes the orientation toward what is yet unknown to the group.

Discussion questions that might be appropriate for this stage might be:

- Are we missing something?
- Who else needs to be here?
- What additional information do we need to have?

Destroying: Signals a willingness to let go of things that are no longer efficient or effective. The triangle-seating configuration signifies that there is a small, targeted group of thought processes, policies, or procedures that need to be replaced in order for the team's work to move forward.

Discussion questions that might be appropriate for this stage might be:

- Which things get in the way of solutions?
- Which elements keep us from moving forward?

Acting: At this point, the team has developed deep listening and analytic skills and an ability to benefit from the collective wisdom of the team. The group might resume a circular seating arrangement and discuss the following questions:

- What is our intent?
- How will we work together?
- How will we support one another?
- How will our work affect the patients, the team, the unit, the organization?

REFLECTION: *Matching Discussions to the Developmental Level of the Team*

It is understood that all groups pass through predictable levels of development. As a result, the most fruitful discussions would be those that addressed issues that were cogent to the developmental level of the group.

How does Wheatley's model for solving complex problems relate to the stages of group development as described by Wheelan?

Appreciative inquiry (AI) is an approach to personal and organizational change which is rooted in positive psychology and based on the belief that the study of what is positive about individuals and systems will help to create positive images and actions in those systems (Cooperrider, Whitney & Stavros, 2008). AI leverages the power of diversity in groups and the infinite relational capacity of human social systems. The energy created by positive inquiry and dialogue generates productive individual and collective action and sustainable success. AI approaches are uniquely suited to interprofessional healthcare teams because their inherent diversity provides opportunities for fruitful conversations, infinite relational possibilities, and innovative action plans.

The practice of AI has conceptual roots in positive psychology and social constructivist theory and is informed by eight essential principles regarding human organizing and change.

1. **The constructionist principle** recognizes the centrality of communication and language to the change process and that reality is an interactive, dialogic construct. The constructionist principle posits that words create worlds.
2. **The simultaneity principle** suggests that change begins at the moment of inquiry.
3. **The poetic principle** suggests that the metaphors and narratives that groups develop can influence the outcome of their collective action.
4. **The anticipatory principle** maintains that positive and hopeful images of the future engender a positive approach to present circumstances. The positive principle proposes

---

REFLECTION: *Personal Appreciative Inquiry*

- Describe a high point in your career as a health professional.
- What particular personal qualities of yours made this possible?
- What is the aspect of your work that makes it most engaging and meaningful for you?
- If you had three wishes for making your work even more engaging and meaningful, what would they be?

that affirmative questions elicit positive affect, which, in turn, provides the energy and engagement required for positive change and growth.

5. **The wholeness principle** states that engaging all stakeholders in a process increases creative alternatives for action and ensures collective investment and engagement.

6. **The enactment principle** claims: *"positive change occurs when the process used to create the change is a living model of the ideal future"* (Whitney et al, 2010, p. 52).

7. **The free-choice principle** suggests that performance improves when individuals are free to work in a manner consistent with their talents and values.

Simply stated, AI is an open, system-wide dialogic approach that focuses on the study of the positive core of an individual, group, or organization. An AI initiative can span from two to three hours to more extended periods of time depending upon the needs of the team or organization. The inclusive nature of AI affords each participant an active voice and an opportunity to dream together and experience their contribution as instrumental in the ongoing creation of a collective vision for the future. The AI process is conceptualized as a four-stage cycle that includes discovery, dream, design, and destiny. This cycle powers the direction for the inquiry and builds a positive foundation upon which human systems can grow and change.

The process begins with the team or organization establishing the topics that they wish to study. Healthcare teams might begin with questions such as: What does this healthcare organization look like when it is at its best? How can the best become the norm? Appropriate AI topics are stated in the affirmative and represent areas about which all constituencies are curious and interested in developing. Topics in healthcare venues might be improving patient care, establishing a relationship-centered organization, fostering wellness behaviors in patients and staff, and increasing the effectiveness of interprofessional teams.

The discovery stage helps participants reflect on their positive core and employs the interviewing of as broad a constituency as possible in order to elucidate the perceived strengths and

STAGE 1: *Discovery*

Appreciative Interview Question (Examples)

- Describe successful interprofessional teams in which you were a member/leader.
- Describe a high point of the team. What did it feel like?
- What did you do to make the team successful?
- What did the members do?
- What individual, group, and organizational resources contribute to the success of the team?
- What are your hopes for this team?

Data from: Cooperrider, Whitney, Starvros (2008). *Appreciative inquiry handbook: for leaders of change.* Brunswick, OH: Crown Custom Publishing.

potentials of the whole team or organization. Interview questions, at this stage, fall into three broad categories that focus on the past, the present, and the future.

During the dream stage, the group is invited to imagine how the best performance can become better. The group uses its collective hope to create positive imagery for the future. Based on the anticipatory principle, it is expected that groups will gravitate toward their co-constructed image of the future. In other words, if the group's self-talk is positive, the likelihood of positive outcomes will be increased. It is crucial that a wide assortment of perspectives inform this dream of the future. There are a variety of ways to unleash the full potential of a group's or organization's imagined future. Whitney et al (2010) provide an example of how a company that managed several long-term care facilities used the dream stage of an appreciative inquiry to create a foundation for a strategic business plan while strengthening a team culture. The group was asked to imagine the world 10 and 20 years into the future when they, personally, were in need of an extended care facility. The group was then asked to address the following questions: What are some of the positive trends in the industry that give you greatest hope for the future of long-term care? Based on those trends, identify six strategic business opportunities that might emerge in the next 10 years. The answers to

STAGE 2: *Dream*

Future Focus Question (Example)
Imagine 10 years into the future.

- What are some of the positive trends in health care that give you the greatest hope for the future of the services that your team provides (e.g., adult rehabilitation services, wellness education, school-based pediatric service)?

- Based on those trends, identify six strategic opportunities for improving patient/client outcomes that might emerge in the next five years.

Data from: Cooperrider, Whitney, Stavros (2008). *Appreciative inquiry handbook: for leaders of change.* Brunswick, OH: Crown Custom Publishing.

those questions served as the basis for design and destiny phases of the AI cycle.

The design stage enables the group to influence its destiny by choosing the opportunities that are most congruent with their collective values and beliefs. The group begins to focus on those aspects of the social architecture—or organizational design elements—that will be targeted. Some components of an interprofessional's social architecture would be vision, purpose, leadership, decision making, communication systems, roles, services, policies, and procedures. One of the key decisions in the

STAGE 3: *Design*

Provocative Proposition (Example)
Design element: Communication
Open and honest communication among all members of the team is essential for efficient and effective healthcare services. All members of the team trust that their input is valued and important and recognize that their active participation is necessary for optimum patient care and outcomes. Meetings are structured to ensure that every member of the team has a voice. Decision-making processes are patient centered and relationship centered.

Data from: Cooperrider, Whitney, Stavros (2008). *Appreciative inquiry handbook: for leaders of change.* Brunswick, OH: Crown Custom Publishing.

design phase is the creation of a positive description of the ideal organization along with propositions regarding how the ideal will be realized. These propositions are stated in the present tense—as if they already exist; they are based on narratives of best practice that were shared in the discovery phase. They transcend current practice and are linked to the aspirations of the group.

The destiny phase allows the participants to establish how they will celebrate their accomplishments and initiate goal-driven action plans and methods for systematically assessing progress. The action plans are informed by the provocative propositions developed in Stage 3. The key questions in Stage 4 are: What are the changes that have occurred as a result of our inquiry? How will we communicate and celebrate the progress we have made? How will we recognize and reward exemplary performance and innovation? What are the time, resources, and personnel needed to support the planned actions, programs, and/or processes?

The need for self-actualization and the need to connect with others are central to the evolutionary process of human systems.

STAGE 4: *Destiny*

Celebrate, Generate, Collaborate for Action (Example)
During your interviews, you heard many stories regarding what makes a successful team.

What were some examples of situations where all members of the team participated in open and honest communication? How were decisions made?

Since we have begun this inquiry, what are some of the positive changes that you have noticed in your team?

What management practices, human resource programs, or work processes would help to make inclusive communication the norm in your team?

What are the time, resources, and personnel that would be required to support and institutionalize these practices?

How will you recognize exemplary performance and progress?

Data from: Cooperrider, Whitney, Stavros (2008). *Appreciative inquiry handbook: for leaders of change.* Brunswick, OH: Crown Custom Publishing.

Teams gain and sustain vitality when leaders and members can find balance between individual and collective needs and focus on a common vision and goals. Consistent positive interactions mitigate workplace stress, facilitate personal renewal, and lay the groundwork for an affirmative, hopeful team-oriented culture. Ever-expanding relational networks increase the self-efficacy of leaders and members and facilitate group development. As teams mature, leadership and responsibility for outcomes become more evenly assumed. The resultant increase in leader and member self-efficacy renders the team more resilient, adaptive, and successful—all of which contribute to the team's overall sustainability. There is no one way for leaders and members to make interprofessional healthcare teams sustainable in the face of change. The path to sustainability of cultures, of organizations, and of teams seems less related to the answers we think we have than the questions we are brave enough to ask. How can we leverage our diverse perspectives? How can we maintain a patient and relationship-centered practice? How can we increase the number, variety, and strength of connections? It is this ongoing process of inquiry that will keep leaders and members of interprofessional healthcare teams operating strategically and effectively in facilitating positive change and growth in themselves and in those whom they aspire to serve.

References

Alvarez-Buylla, A., & Temple, S. (1998). *Journal of Neurobiology, 36*(2), 105–110.

Bandler, R., & Grinder, J. (1975). *The structure of magic, volume II: A Book about communication and change.* Palo Alto, CA: Science and Behavior Books.

Boyatzis, R., & McKee, A. (2005). *Resonant leadership.* Boston, MA: Harvard Business School Press.

Briskin, A., Erickson, S., Ott, J., & Callanan, T. (2009). *The power of collective wisdom and the trap of collective folly.* San Francisco, CA: Berrett-Koehler.

Clarke, D. (2010). Achieving teamwork in stroke units: The contribution of opportunistic dialogue. *Journal of Interprofessional Care, 24*(3), 285–297.

Cooperrider, D., Whitney, D., & Stavros, J. (2008). *Appreciative inquiry handbook: For leaders of change.* Brunswick, OH: Crown Custom Publishing.

Dickerson, S. & Kemeny, M. (2004). Acute stressors and cortisol responses: A theoretical integration and synthesis of laboratory research. *Psychological Bulletin, 130,* 355–391.

Diener, E., & Lucas, R. (2000). Subjective emotional well-being. In M. Lewis & J. Haviland-Jones (Eds.), *Handbook of emotion* (2nd ed., pp. 325–337). New York, NY: Guilford.

Diener, E., Suh, E., Lucas, R., & Smith, H. (1999). Subjective well-being: Three decades of progress. *Psychological Bulletin, 125,* 276–302.

Dilts, R. (1999). *Sleight of mouth: The magic of conversational belief change.* Capitola, CA: Meta Publishers.

Ekman, P. (1997). Should we call it expression or communication? *Innovation in Social Science Research, 10,* 333–344.

Ekman, P., Camps, J., Davidson, R. & de Waal, F. (Eds.). (2003). Emotions Inside out: 130 Years after Darwin's The Expression of the Emotions in Man and Animals. *Annals of the New York Academy of Sciences, Volume 1000.* New York, NY: New York Academy of Sciences.

Ekman, P. (2004). *Emotions revealed: Recognizing faces and feelings to improve communication and emotional life* (2nd ed.). New York, NY: Henry Holt.

Frederickson, B. (2003, July–August). The value of positive emotions. *American Scientist, 91,* 330–335.

Frederickson, B. (2009). *Positivity.* New York, NY: Crown.

Goleman, D. (2003). *Destructive emotions: A scientific dialogue with the* Dalai Lama. New York, NY: Bantam Books.

Gottman, J., Levenson, R., & Woodin, E. (2001). Facial expression during marital conflict. *Journal of Family Communication, 1*(2001), 37–57

Hall, L., & Bodenhammer, B. (2002). *Mind lines: Lines for changing minds.* Clifton, CO: NeuroSematic Publications.

Hamm, A., Schupp, H., & Weike, A. (2003). Motivational organization of emotions: Autonomic changes, cortical responses, and reflex modulation. In R. J. Davidson, K. R. Sherer, & H., H. Goldsmith (Eds.), *The handbook of affective sciences* (pp. 187–211). Oxford, England: University Press.

Hatfield, E., Cacioppo, J. T., & Rapson, R. L. (1993). *Emotional contagion*. New York, NY: Cambridge University Press.

Landro, L. (2012, January 3). When nurses catch compassion fatigue, patients suffer. *The Wall Street Journal*, http://online.wsj.com

Langer, E., & Imber, L. (1979). When practice makes imperfect: The debilitating effects of overlearning. *Journal of Personality and Social Psychology, 37*, 2014–2025.

Lewis, T., Amini, F., & Lannon, R. (2000). *A general Theory of love*. New York, NY: Random House.

Ludema, J. (2001). From deficit discourse to vocabularies of hope: The power of appreciation. In D. Cooperrider, P. Sorensen, Jr., T. Yaeger, & D. Whitney (Eds.), *Appreciative Inquiry: An emerging direction for organizational development* (pp. 443–466). Champaign, IL: Stipes Publishing.

McEwen, B. (1998). Protective and damaging effects of stress mediators. *New England Journal of Medicine, 338*, 171–179.

McMurtry, A. (2007). Reinterpreting interdisciplinary health teams from a complexity science perspective. *University of Alberta Health Sciences Journal, 4*(1), 33–42.

Sapolsky, R. (2004). *Why zebras Don't get ulcers* (3rd ed.). New York, NY: Harper Collins.

Segerstom, S., & Miller, G. (2004). Psychological stress and the human immune system: Ameta-analytic study of 30 years of inquiry. *Psychological Bulletin, 130*(4), 601–630.

Strazdins, L. (2000). Emotional work and emotional contagion. In N. Ashkanasy, W. Zerbe, & C. Hartel (Eds.), *Emotions in the workplace: Research, theory and practice* (pp. 232–250). Westport, CT: Quorum Books.

Wheatley, M. (2005). *Finding our Way: Leadership for an uncertain Time*. San Francisco, CA: Berrett-Koehler Publishers, Inc.

Wheelan, S., Burchill, C., & Tilin, F. (2003). The link between teamwork and patients' outcomes in intensive care units. *American Journal of Critical Care, 12,* 527–534.

Whitney, D., Trosten-Bloom, A., Radu, K. (2010). *Appreciative leadership: Focus on what works to drive winning performance.* New York, NY: McGraw-Hill.

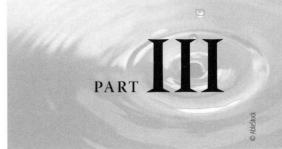

Building and Sustaining Collaborative Interprofessional Teams Activities

Activity 1: Mini 360-Degree Feedback Exercise

While self-reflection is an essential leadership behavior, you need to establish whether your view of yourself is consistent with those who you aspire to influence. A 360-degree perspective allows you to find out how you are viewed by your superiors, your coworkers, and your subordinates. Ask them the following questions regarding your effectiveness as a leader/member of a team. How do their answers compare to the answers you would give about yourself?

Similar answers will highlight areas of strength while discrepancies will provide clues regarding areas for improvement.

- What should I do more of?
- What should I do less of?
- What could I do to contribute more positively to the team?

Activity 2: The Art of Culture

Culture can seem like a difficult concept to grasp yet we all know that each team (or organization) has a unique feel. This exercise helps you capture the feeling of your team (or organization) by drawing a picture of how you see it now and depicting your vision for a collaborative, interdisciplinary, patient-centered culture for the future.

1. Think about how it feels to work where you work. Write some adjectives or short phrases that describe your culture and/or a metaphor that you have used that describes the culture.
2. Draw a picture of the current culture of your team or organization as it feels to you now.
3. Now think about how you would like the culture to be in the next 3–5 years. Write some adjectives or short phrases that describe your culture and/or a metaphor that you have used that describes the culture.
4. Draw a picture of the new culture.
5. Look at the two pictures. What do you think can be done to help change this culture? What is something you can change about your own behavior or attitude that may facilitate this change? How can you influence others to work towards positive culture change in your organization?

Activity 3: Checklist of Behaviors That Foster a Collaborative Culture

Check each item that applies to your team. The headings that have the most checks will indicate team strengths while those with the least checks will indicate opportunities for improvement. How can you facilitate a collaborative interprofessional team culture?

Role and Goal Clarification	
Encourages the process of goal, role, task clarification	
Supports division of labor necessary to accomplish group goals	
Communicates in Order to Achieve Team Goals	
Encourages the adoption of an open communication structure where all member input and feedback is heard	
Promotes an appropriate ratio of the group task and members' emotional engagement and group process	
Promotes the use of affirmative dialogue	
Encourages use of effective conflict management strategies	
Employs effective problem-solving and decision-making procedures	
Develops Collaborative Team Norms	
Encourages the establishment of norms that support productivity, innovation, and freedom of expression	
Discourages any group tendency to overlegislate individual behavior through the adoption of excessive or unnecessary rules	
Individuals voluntarily conform with norms that promote group effectiveness	
Welcomes diverse perspectives	
Takes Personal Responsibility for the Team's Success	
Members commit to personal and professional development	
Members remain current in their respective fields	
Members actively draw on each other's expertise	
Members promote cohesion and cooperation	

Members take a positive approach to seeking solutions for the team's problems	
Members interact with others outside of the team in ways that promote the team's ability to interface within the larger organizational context	
Members have an understanding of group development and group process	
Employ Energizing Strategies	
Moves toward relationship building	
Engages team members on a personal level	
Makes time for reflection and personal renewal	
Stays appreciative and positive; discovers opportunities in challenges	

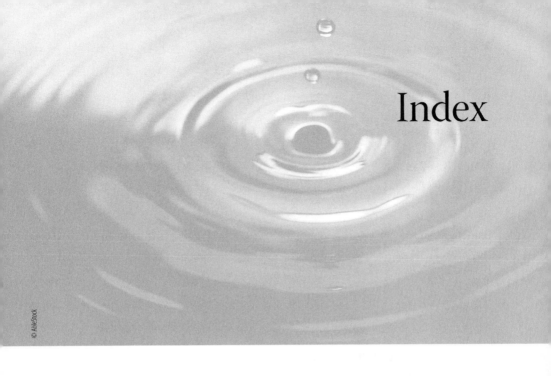

Index

A

Accommodating learning style, 104
Achievement motive/need, 97
Action oriented roles, 43, 44
Adjourning, 25
Adult/andragogy learning, 100–101, 112
Affiliation motive/need, 97
Affirmative dialogue, 191–193
Alderfer, C. P., 5
Anticipatory principle, 198–199
Appreciative inquiry
    principles of, 198–199
    stages of, 199–203
Artifacts, 154
Assimilating learning style, 104
Austill-Clausen, R., 181–184

B

Basic assumption group, 23
Belbin, R., 43, 44–45
Benne, K., 42–43
Big five theory, 79
Bion, W., 22–23, 24
Blake, R., 80–81
Blanchard, K., 79, 80
Boyatzis, R., 88
Briggs, K. C., 72–79

C

Catalysts, leaders as, 110, 114–115
Circles of life exercise, 131–132
Coaches, leaders as, 110, 112–113
Cocreative power, 96
Coercive power, 95
Cognitive tasks, 143–144
Collaborative culture
    See also Culture
    activities, 157–158, 209–211
    Austill-Clausen's views, 182–183
    behaviors that foster, 210–211
    Fox's and Kurilko's views, 165–166
    importance of, 155
    Keshner's views, 174–175
    Kirby's views, 178
    questions to guide, 156
    Sinnott's views, 160–162
    Verrillo's views, 169–170
Collective resonance, 21
Communication
    diversity, recognizing and respecting, 56
    feedback, 54
    hierarchical, problem with, 54
    Johari window, 49–52
    learning styles compared with styles of, 46–49

Communication *(Cont.)*
    networks, 52–53
Community
    focus, goals, and methods of, 12
    of practice, 157
Conflict, managing, 145–147, 150
Conscious group, unconscious versus, 22–23
Constructionist principle, 198
Contingency theories, 79–81
Converging learning style, 104
Conversations, dynamic, 9
Counterdependency/fight (stage II), 29–30, 31
Culture
    See also Collaborative culture
    activity, 209
    analyzing team, 184
    cues, 154
    defined, 153–154

D

Davidson, B., 33–34
Deep-level (psychological) diversity, 139–140
Deep listening, 143
Demographic diversity, 139
Dependency, 23, 24
Dependency/inclusion (stage I), 28–29, 31
Design stage, 201–202
Destiny stage, 202
Discovery stage, 199–200
Diverging learning style, 104
Diversity
    categories, 137, 138
    conflict, managing, 145–147, 150
    deep-level (psychological), 139–140
    dimensions of, 138
    guidelines for managing, 149
    integrating the levels of, 140–144

Diversity *(Cont.)*
   recognizing and respecting, 56
   surface-level (demographic), 139
Dream stage, 200–201

E

Ecologists, leaders as, 110, 115–116
Edmondson, A., 9, 33
Ely, R. J., 140
Emotional intelligence
   checklist, 84–87
   development of, 82–83
   domains, 83
Emotions, responses to, 189
Empowerment, 115–116
Enactment principle, 199
Expert power, 95

F

Feedback, 54, 209
Fiedler, F., 79
Fight-flight, 23, 24
Fisher, R., 146
Follett, M. P., 96
Forming, 25, 26
Fox, T., 163–166
Free-choice principle, 199
French, J., 95
Fundamental Interpersonal Relations Orientation (FIRO), 99

G

Garman, A., 117
Goals
   group, 41–42

Goals *(Cont.)*
    SMART, 66–68, 133–134
Goleman, D., 82–83
Gray, B., 115, 143
Group development
    activities, 63–68
    model of, 26–27
    size and productivity, impact of, 34–35
    termination, 33
    time needed for, 36–37
Group development, stages of
    counterdependency/fight (stage II), 29–30,
        31
    dependency/inclusion (stage I), 28–29, 31
    identifying, 27–33
    role of, 23, 25–26
    team productivity and, 33–34
    time needed at each stage, 36–37
    trust/structure (stage III), 30, 31, 32
    work/productivity (stage IV), 30, 31, 32
Group Development Questionnaire (GDQ), 26
Group life
    basic assumption, 23
    environment/context, 23
    experiences, 23, 24
    group as a unit, 22
    individual members, 22
    unconscious versus conscious, 22–23
    work, 22, 23, 24
Groups
    cultural differences, 19
    defined, 5
    difference between teams and, 5–7
    focus, goals, methods of, 11
    goals, 41–42
    identification of, 6
    I/We perspective, 20
    norms, 21, 39–41
    roles, 3–4, 42–46
    systems approach to, 7–15

H

Health care teams, future of
   Austill-Clausen's views, 184
   Fox's and Kurilko's views, 166
   Keshner's views, 176
   Kirby's views, 180
   Sinnott's views, 163
   Verrillo's views, 171–172
Hegel, 7
Hersey, P., 79, 80
Human Side of Enterprise, The (McGregor), 94

I

Individuals, focus, goals and methods of, 11
Institutes of Medicine, 54
Interpersonal, focus, goals, and methods, 11
Interpretations, 191
Interprofessional teams
   activities, 209–211
   Austill-Clausen's views, 181–184
   Fox's and Kurilko's views, 163–166
   Keshner's views, 172–176
   Kirby's views, 177–180
   Sinnott's views, 158–163
   Verrillo's views, 168–172
I/We perspective, 20

J

Johari window, 49–52
Jung, C., 73

K

Kahn, R., 7
Katz, D., 7

Katzenbach, J. R., 5–6
Keshner, E., 172–176
Kirby, J. J., 176–180
Kolb, D., 101–104, 112
Kolb Learning Style Inventory (LSI), 102–104
Kurilko, R., 163–166

L

Leaders, attitudes needed by, 110
Leaders, roles and skills of
    catalyst, 110, 114–115
    coach, 110, 112–113
    ecologist, 110, 115–116
    learner, 110, 111–112
    partner, 110, 114
Leadership
    activities, 123–134
    big five theory, 79
    contingency and situational theories and, 79–81
    emotional intelligence, 82–87
    grid, 80–81
    Myers-Briggs Type Indicator (MBTI), 72–78, 123–125
    personality/trait theories and, 72–79
    perspectives on, 72
    positional, 72, 80
    relational theories, 82
    resonant, 87–89
    styles, summary of, 99
Leadership building blocks
    learning, 100–105
    motivation, 97–100
    power, 94–97
Learners
    leaders as, 110, 111–112
    teams as, 195–203
Learning and learning styles
    accommodating, 104
    adult/andragogy, 100–101, 112

Learning and learning styles *(Cont.)*
    assimilating, 104
    communication styles compared with, 46–49
    converging, 104
    diverging, 104
    Kolb Learning Style Inventory (LSI), 102–104
    meaning perspective, 101
    self-directed, 101
Leavitt, H., 52
Legitimate power, 95
Levi, R., 21
Lewin, K., 42
Lifeline exercise, 126, 127
Listening, deep, 143

M

Mannix, E., 137, 138
McClelland, D., 97, 98
McGregor, D., 94
McKee, A., 88
McMurtry, A., 195
Meaning perspective, 101
Mezirow, J., 101
Motivation, 97–100
    values and, 129–130
Moulton, J., 80–81
Myers, I. B., 72–79
Myers-Briggs Type Indicator (MBTI), 72–78, 123–125

N

Neale, M. A., 137, 138
Negotiations, 146
Nembhard, I., 9, 33
Networks, communication, 52–53
Nonverbal clues, responses to, 189
Norming, 25, 26
Norms, 21, 39–41

O

Objective criteria, 145–146
Open systems theory, 7–8
Organizational culture, 8–9
Organizational roles, 42
Organizations, focus, goals and methods of, 12

P

Pairing, 23, 24
Partners, leaders as, 110, 114
People oriented roles, 43, 44–45
Performing, 25, 26
Personality/trait theories
    big five theory, 79
    Myers-Briggs Type Indicator (MBTI), 72–78
Personal renewal, importance of, 189–190
Poetic principle, 198
Positional leadership, 72, 80
Power, 94–97
Power motive/need, 97–98
Problem solving, behaviors needed for, 195–196
Problem solving stages
    acting, 197
    cooling/quieting, 196
    destroying, 197
    enriching, 196
    magnetizing, 196–197
Procedural tasks, 143
Psychological diversity, 139–140

R

Radu, K., 116
Raven, B., 95
Referent power, 95
Reframing, 193–194

Relational theories, 82
Relationship management, 83, 86–87
Resonance, 188
Resonant leaders, 87–89
Ringelman, M., 34
Roberts, L. M., 140
Roles, 3–4, 42–46

S

Sacrifice syndrome, 189
Schein, E., 153–154
Self-awareness, 83, 84
Self-efficacy, 155
Self-management, 83, 84–85, 187–188
Sheats, P., 42–43
Simultaneity principle, 198
Sinnott, M., 158–163
Situational theories, 79–81
Skillman, R., 110
Sluyter, D., 7–8
SMART goals, 66–68, 133–134
Smith, D. K., 5–6
Social awareness, 83, 85–86
Social brain, 20
Social loafing, 34
Socioemotional or maintenance roles, 42
Storming, 25, 26
Structural tasks, 144
Studer, Q., 145
Suchman, A., 7–8
Surface-level (demographic) diversity, 139
Sustainable systems
    affirmative dialogue, 191–193
    appreciative inquiry, 198–203
    examples of, 188
    personal renewal, importance of, 189–190
    reframing, 193–194
    self-management, 187–188

Systems theory
    applications, 10–15
    case study, 12–14
    development of, 7
    groups and, 7–10

T

Task roles, 42
Teams
    See also Health care teams, future of; Interprofessional teams
    difference between groups and, 5–7
    as learners, 195–203
    need for, 4
    productivity and group development stage, 33–34
Termination, 33
Theory X, 94
Theory Y, 94
Thought oriented roles, 43, 44
Tilin, F., 33–34
TOPS (Team Orientation and Performance Survey), 63–66
Trosten-Bloom, A., 116
Trust/structure (stage III), 30, 31, 32
Tuckman, B., 25–26
Turnover, staff, 141–142

U

Unconscious versus conscious group, 22–23
Ury, W., 146

V

Values, 126, 128–130, 154
Verrillo, S. C., 167–172
von Bertanffly, L., 7

W

Wenger, E., 157
Wheatley, M., 156, 195
Wheelan, S., 26–34, 35, 42
Whitney, D., 116, 200
Wholeness principle, 199
Williams, 27
Williamson, P., 7–8
Work group, 22, 23, 24
Work/productivity (stage IV), 30, 31, 32

Y

Yukl, G. A., 97–98

Z

Zeitgeist theory, 72
Zolno, S., 110, 154